Bravery

by
Kim Gemmell

First Edition –December 2012

ISBN
978-1-4602-0609-6 (Hardcover)
978-1-4602-0607-2 (Paperback)
978-1-4602-0608-9 (eBook)

Produced by:

FriesenPress

Suite 300 – 852 Fort Street
Victoria, BC, Canada V8W 1H8

www.friesenpress.com

Distributed to the trade by The Ingram Book Company
Cover design: Pixelgems, Chilliwack, BC
Cover photo: Penelope Ball
Editor: Edward Strauss

I wish to dedicate Bravery to my beautiful and miraculous son, Avery. This book would not exist if you had not been born to me. I love you more than life, my little monkey man!

Dorothy!
Thanks for sharing
in our journey!
Love,
Kim

Contents

Chapter 1
A White Picket Fence

Life can sure throw some curve balls at you every now and again. I've certainly had my share, and I guess a good way to start my story is by saying that Friday, May 29, 1998 marked the beginning of the most surreal time of my life and started me on my tumultuous journey. Before I begin to tell my story, however, I feel I should let you know who I am, as well as introduce you to the amazing people who helped me through such trying times. It's important to give you some insight into my family, because they are the people who built the foundation of who I am and provided me with the values and courage that kept me going through such a harrowing time.

I was born and raised in the small town of Chilliwack just outside of Vancouver in British Columbia, Canada. I consider myself fortunate to have had nurturing parents who provided me with an exceptional childhood filled with wonderful memories. I had some great friends, but most of my time was spent riding my horse on Grandma's farm. I have always been a huge animal lover. Some people would joke with me that I liked animals more than people. There was probably some truth to that, yet, as I grew so did my social life.

Probably my strongest asset was my optimism and positive outlook about life. I did at times display a strong will, and on the rare occasion, when provoked, my Irish temper would emerge. For the most part, however, I was a happy-go-lucky person who loved to laugh and have fun. I was known as a bit of a prankster, but generally stayed out of trouble thanks to my parents, whose unconditional love and support guided me to make good choices.

Empathy is one of the traits that I value most. I consider myself a compassionate person, and always tried to help people in need. In school I often befriended the kids who were having a hard time fitting in. I despised bullies, and felt compelled to stick up for anyone getting teased. I didn't realize how much it was appreciated until my ten-year grad reunion. At least five or six people came up to me that night and told me how much it meant to them that I had supported them in school. I was most honored to hear this.

I had a few boyfriends along the way, but it wasn't until I moved to Vancouver in my early twenties that I met my future husband, Cam Gemmell. He was going to university, working part time as a waiter at a popular restaurant. I was going to school taking a marketing program, and working part time at the health club beside the restaurant where he worked. We met through mutual friends and our relationship started as a friendship. Mom and Dad would often visit and take me out for dinner where Cam worked. No matter where we sat, it always seemed that Cam was our waiter. Mom noticed and often said, "I think this guy has a big crush on you." (Cam later told me he bribed the waiters to switch sections so he could serve us.)

One evening, a few friends and I went to the restaurant after work. Cam had just finished his shift and was sitting down having a drink with a couple of friends. They asked if we wanted to join them, and we said, "Sure." Cam turned to me to start up a conversation, and that's when I knew. I looked into his eyes and for some reason something changed. I saw him in a different way. I felt like I had just drunk a glass of hot chocolate: my stomach tingled, my heart felt warm, and I knew that this was it.

I don't know why it had taken so long for me to fall for him. It was suddenly so apparent what a wonderful person he was—a kind, sensitive man who always brought a smile to my face. Not only did he have a great sense of humor, but he was very attractive, standing six foot two with bright blue eyes, full lips that I just wanted to kiss, and light golden-brown, wavy hair. He kind of reminded me of a California surfer boy. Most importantly, his values and morals set him apart from any other guy I had dated.

We soon found ourselves spending most of our time together, never wanting to be apart. Within a year we were engaged then we married the following year in October, 1991.

We were having the time of our lives. Blessed with many great friends, we were always on the go, whether it was skiing at Whistler, or just hanging out in the lounge at the athletic club playing pool with our friends. At the time I couldn't have asked for anything more.

As it often does when you're having fun, time flew by, and before we knew it a few years had passed. The time came to discuss adding to our little family. We owned a two-bedroom townhouse, had a bit of money in the bank, and had already spent close to four great years together. All the signs pointed us to the next step, and we were ready. Within a month of talking about starting a family, I became pregnant. We were very excited, but at the same time a little nervous about this new life that we were embarking on.

We were both very busy working full time. I was in sales as an account executive with a major beauty supply company, and Cam was in sales with a waste management company. Both our territories were closer to the Valley (as people here call the lower Fraser River Valley outside Vancouver) so it made sense to move back to Chilliwack. Real estate was much more affordable and my mom offered to baby-sit for me after my maternity leave was over. Mom and Dad were thrilled that we were moving back. So we sold our townhouse in Vancouver and bought a much bigger home in Chilliwack for a lot less money. Things seemed to be falling into place perfectly. My pregnancy felt great for the most part, and I only gained about fifteen pounds, even though I ate constantly.

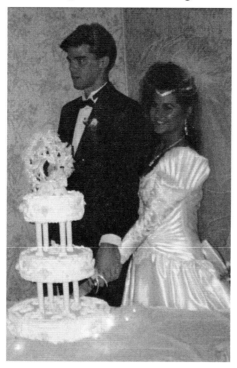

(Cam and I cutting our wedding cake)

Chapter 2
It Doesn't Get Better Than This

On February 9, 1995, our wonderful little girl Jesse arrived in our lives. However, it took seventeen hours of agonizing labor filled with the most horrendous pain imaginable. I wasn't sure who looked worse, Cam or me. He was white as a ghost because he thought I was dying. I ripped every one of his belt loops off his jeans by putting my fingers through them and tugging frantically, and the collar of his T-shirt was stretched down past his chest.

Although I swore never to give birth to another child, Jesse was worth every minute of the pain. She was three weeks early but a healthy 5.6 pounds. I know all parents think their newborn is the most gorgeous baby, however, no one could have told me that Jesse wasn't the most beautiful baby ever. She looked like a little cherubic porcelain doll with big blue eyes and perfectly-defined features.

I felt extremely blessed with life. Jesse was the ideal baby, barely ever crying and nursing almost every two hours around the clock. I didn't mind because she was growing so fast. Other than feeling like a full time milking machine and being a little sleep-deprived, I was delighted with how things were going.

Looking back, I find most of our first few months of parenting quite comical. We were such novices. We had no idea what we were doing. We had never been around babies and were amongst the first of our friends to have children. I have a video of Cam changing Jesses' first diaper; it took him twelve minutes. Jesse left the hospital in her first cute little knitted outfit—on backwards. (My fault.) However, it didn't take long for us to become a great team.

I was a little surprised that I fit into the role of motherhood so naturally. I'm sure much of that was because everything was so easy with Jesse. She was a happy baby full of smiles, and we were the typical proud parents. Cam was the best dad, rushing home every day to spend time with Jesse. I could tell she was going to have her father's sense of humor. I loved watching the two of them. Cam would pretend to bang himself against the wall and then fall down. Jesse would laugh hysterically with her contagious belly laugh.

After Cam and I moved back to Chilliwack, I spent most of my spare time with my best friend, Tracee. We'd known each other since we were young kids in school, and when I moved back to Chilliwack our friendship rekindled. Tracee had married Len Kentala, a very down-to-earth guy who reminded me a little of Cam. Her second son, Brett, was only a couple months younger than Jesse, so we had a lot in common. We were both on maternity leave and we would often get together at each others' houses, as well as spending many afternoons shopping.

I was just as close to Tracee's sister Nikcole, who was two years younger than her. She had moved to Vancouver shortly before me to attend post-secondary school. When I lived in Vancouver we had hung out a lot. In fact, I was the one who introduced her to my friend Rob, who later became her husband. On many weekends Nikcole and Rob would drive out to Chilliwack and spend time with us. They were expecting their first child shortly after Jesse was born.

Up to this point, my life was pretty full and I had no complaints. I guess if there was one content, happy point in my life that I would have chosen to freeze-frame, this would have been it. I hadn't a worry in the world. I had wonderful people in my life and I felt so fortunate to have an amazing family who had given me all the love and values I needed to be a great mom.

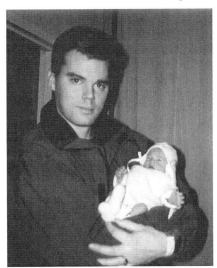 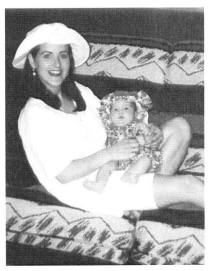

(Cam holding Jesse the day she was born) (Mom and Jesse at four months)

Chapter 3
Pillars Of Support

Now that I've explained where I was at in life, it's important to tell you about the incredible family members whose support I couldn't have done without. If it hadn't been for them I don't think I would have been able to cope with the nearly impossible circumstances that came my way.

I'll start with one of the most incredible people I have met or ever will meet, my maternal grandmother, Gwen McKay. Many of my values came from her, and a large part of who I am is because of her influence on my life. Even though she's not with us anymore she plays a very important part in this book. Unfortunately, she died of a heart attack at age sixty-nine, soon after I moved to Vancouver. This was one of the biggest loses of my life. I had loved being around her, and didn't feel she had finished teaching me all of her valuable life lessons. Granted, in the twenty-two years I was lucky enough to have had with her, I did learn plenty. Grandma lived on a forty-acre farm just down the road from us, and we were very close, spending almost every weekend together.

She was a most unique woman. She was not only strikingly beautiful, but she carried the most wonderful presence about her. It was apparent where my mom got her good looks from. They looked a lot alike, sharing the same highly-arched eyebrows that perfectly framed their kind blue eyes, and prominent cheek bones that highlighted their beautiful olive skin. Grandma had a healthy chubbiness, like a grandma should have, and always wore a bright smile that made her eyes twinkle even more.

Grandma had only one leg, but it never slowed her down, and I think in some ways it enriched her life. Years earlier, in the 1950s when Grandma was in her thirties, she had been in town running some errands, and had stopped to talk to a friend sitting in her parked car. Two cars that were drag racing crashed into each other and then into my Grandma on the sidewalk. The only way anyone was able to find her was because a little piece of her dress was peeking out from underneath one of the smashed cars. She was almost dead, and her right leg was crushed and bleeding profusely. My mom, who was fifteen at the time, had been waiting in their car for her. She had seen the entire accident but sat frozen with shock. She thought her mom was dead.

The police arrived at the scene quickly, and one officer walked up to Grandma's car and asked if there was a Barby McKay there. My mom responded, "That's me." The officer then explained that the lady who had been hit was calling out for her. Scared out of her wits, she ran to Grandma, who was lying on the sidewalk. Covered in blood and barely coherent she looked up at her daughter and said, "Now don't you worry, Barby … I'm going to be fine … I won't leave you."

Soon after, the ambulance came and rushed Grandma to the hospital. Grandpa, my Mom, and her brother Jim and sister Geraldine, paced the hospital floor hoping and praying Grandma would be okay. The doctors hadn't placed much hope on her survival because they couldn't stop the blood flow, and she had already lost a large amount. Then the news came that there was a chance Grandma would live, but had to have her leg amputated. A blood clot had formed in the leg that had been crushed, and that's what saved her life. The doctors said it was nothing short of a miracle.

I am so grateful my Grandma lived through that horrible accident; the life lessons I learned from her were invaluable. She always said to me, "Appreciate every day because you don't know what tomorrow brings." She had learned that lesson firsthand, the hard way. I also clearly remember her telling me, "I never realized what a privilege it was to have both my legs, and the freedom of being able to hop on my bike and feel the wind against my face. Life is full of little precious things that many overlook."

A lot of her wisdom went over my head when I was a kid, but as time went on I understood her much better. I learned to be thankful for subtleties like the smile I would get from the smell of fresh-cut grass, or the simple pleasure of feeling the warmth of the sun on my face.

One of Grandma's favorite sayings was, "You are only as beautiful on the outside as you are on the inside." I really believed it, so I tried to always be beautiful on the inside because I wanted to be just like my grandma.

Many weekends I woke at Grandma's house with the delicious aroma of bacon, eggs, and homemade pancakes cooking on the griddle. It was quite remarkable how she flew around the kitchen on her little stool with wheels. It never failed: no matter how nice or rainy it was outside she would say to me, "Oh, Kimmi! Look outside. What a beautiful day it is. Listen to the birds singing." I didn't get it until much later in life. Now I always listen for the birds and appreciate their song. To me, Grandma lives on in the songs of the birds.

Grandma would go to bed much later than I because she was always busy baking for people or making someone a special cake, but she always lay down with me as we recited our evening prayers. Many years later when I was an adolescent, Grandma told me how she had gotten such a kick out of our prayers. She said, "I would begin, 'Now I lay me down to sleep,' then proceed with many "Thank You's" and requests for God to protect everyone and to keep them safe, then all of a sudden you would chime in, 'And please God, bring Jesus back down to Earth so He can help all the people who need it.'" Grandma said that I made this request *every* prayer without fail. She said this is how she knew my faith in the Lord was sincere.

Yes, I spent a lot of time at Grandma's, much of it riding my horse around her farm. I would always find four-leaf clovers, sometimes even while I was on my horse. Grandma thought I was very special because of that. She said she had never found a four-leaf clover in her entire life. I was a teenager, and had found probably over thirty. It wasn't until many years later, after the birth of my son, that I came to attach a greater significance to my clover discoveries.

Grandma's eccentricities showed up in many ways, but mostly when she took all seven grandchildren out for fun. For our Friday night entertainment we would often all pack into the old station wagon and park outside the local drinking establishment to watch the drunken people stagger out and fall down. It was also her way of teaching us to never abuse alcohol or drugs. We kids thought it was an amusing way to learn a valuable lesson.

On most Sundays, Grandma would pick us up and take us to Sunday school. I looked forward to the service, but not as much as what we usually did *after* the service. Grandma was quite the antique collector, so often after church we would go see what treasures we could find at the garbage dump. My brother Steven and I found lots of neat stuff, much to the chagrin of my mom.

Once in a while Grandma took all of us grandchildren to stay at a hotel in Vancouver. She didn't have a lot of money so the lodgings left a little to be desired. One time we saw two men fighting on the street outside our hotel in East Vancouver. We ended up helping one of the men look for his tooth on the sidewalk. It's kind of crazy when I think about those times now, but oh, how much fun it was! Those were some of my best memories.

I also remember Grandma's enormous generosity. At least once a week she would spend hours in the kitchen of her old farmhouse cooking and baking. Then she'd take it to her friends who didn't have much money. I will never forget what she did for our neighbor, 'Little John,' who lived in an old rundown shack beside her. He was getting pretty old and Grandma would always check in on him and give him some baking. After some years, he got a pretty severe case of dementia and couldn't take care of himself anymore. He had no living family members, so (not surprisingly) Grandma took him in. She had a spare room in her house, and that became his home.

He mostly slept and watched TV, but once in a while he would feel up for a walk. One of us grandchildren would have to go too to make sure he didn't get lost. Grandma took very good care of Little John for the next couple years, until the day he had to go to the hospital. He became quite ill, and Grandma could no longer take care of him. He kept calling out "Momma, Momma" as the paramedics wheeled him away. I think he made it three days in the hospital before he died.

I am most privileged to have known such a woman as Gwen McKay, and not many days have gone by since her passing that I don't think about her.

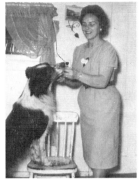
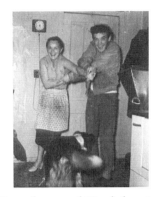

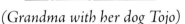
(Grandma with her dog Tojo)   (Grandma and Dad dancing)

My mom, a former beauty queen who won the title of Miss Chilliwack in 1959, had a generous heart as well. She was just as beautiful on the inside as she was on the outside. Whenever people have told me that I look just like her, I've been very flattered. Mom has always looked very young for her age, and her hourglass figure invited stares wherever she went. Her one and only love, however, was Dad. They had been together since she was fourteen years old. Dad hadn't had a very good mother or home life, and had left home at fifteen, so Grandma invited him to live with them. She took him in and that's where he stayed until Mom and he got married and they built their own house.

My memories of her consist of many fun stories about their escapades when they were young. I loved it when Mom told stories about their younger days; her eyes twinkled as she spoke with spirited enthusiasm and precise detail, leaving the impression it had happened just last week. One of my favorites was how Dad fell off the stairs at the Coliseum when it was announced that Mom had won the Miss Chilliwack beauty pageant.

He was always extremely proud to be her husband, and his adoring looks were apparent. One of the many ways he showed his devotion was by spoiling her with the biggest diamond rings I had ever seen. All through the years they remained as close as they were when they had met. Theirs was such a rare love.

She was just as great a mom as she was a wife. Her unconditional love and support meant more to me than she will ever know. It would have been impossible to have been more loved by her. Mom was a real softy. All my friends said that I was spoiled to death. I never wanted to admit it, but they were probably right. Not many kids had a horse when they were five. However, I was always very appreciative of my parents' generosity, and tried to never take anything for granted.

Because of my mom, I was able to grow to become a happy, well-adjusted person who always felt wanted and loved. Everybody who knows her has only nice things to say about her. She is a very positive person, who taught me that I could achieve anything I wanted to. There is no such word as "can't" in her vocabulary, and she always told me that as well.

She spent a lot of her time taking me to horse shows in my youth. I rode competitively, and it was a very busy lifestyle, and quite expensive. Much of her effort would be making sure I had all I needed to excel. I had a great horse trainer and usually did well, but no matter how I placed in any of my shows, Mom always expressed how proud she was of me. She had the ability to always make me feel good and cheer me up, even after a bad day. The confidence and self esteem she instilled in me has served me well in life. I have come through many challenging times still in one piece and standing tall because of the strength she gave me.

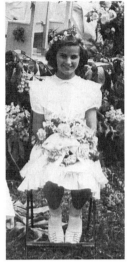
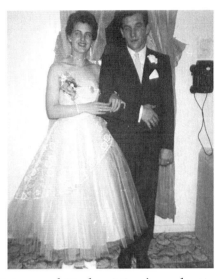

(Mom, Miss May Queen)   (Mom and Dad at Mom's graduation)

My dad was not a big man, but he was ruggedly handsome with very prominent, sharp features and a fit physique. He never went unnoticed when he walked into a room; his piercing green eyes had a way of captivating people. He was a tough guy, yet possessed a very kind soul. He too was a real softy, especially when it came to me, his little girl – but also toward others.

Dad owned his own trucking company and the flag girls told me how he would give them his lunch when they didn't have any, and he would give away his water and juice to the asphalt workers on very hot days.

He was a treasure, but oh, he surely had an Irish temper. You never wanted to be the guy who had done him wrong. In his youth he got into many street fights. He then turned to pro boxing, winning the Lightweight Golden Gloves Championship.

(Dad walking down the sidewalk after competing in a boxing match.)

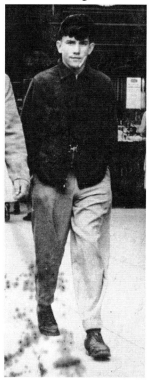

There was no doubt he was a tough guy. I remember being worried I wouldn't find a man who would meet with Dad's approval. Fortunately, he liked Cam right off the bat and knew he was a good guy who would treat me with respect.

Dad was always so concerned about my welfare. When I was a teenager he told my friend Nikcole and I and I not to have children. He said, "Once you have kids, you'll spend the rest of your life worrying about them." It wasn't until much later in life when we had our own children that we began to understand what he meant. He was trying to spare us the pain and heartaches that come with the job. Nikcole and I still chuckle about that remark, especially when we're going through the challenges that sometimes come with parenting.

Dad's remark turned out to be quite funny in another sense because once my daughter Jesse came into his world he was completely captivated. Jesse and he had a relationship like none other. She was the only person who could get my dad to stop whatever he was doing and play with her for hours. Grandpa and Grandma's house was the place she wanted to be. We would go there for a visit several times a week and Jesse couldn't get out of the car fast enough to run and give them a big hug.

It was truly remarkable watching Jesse's face light up when she was around Grandpa. The two of them would often hang out outside, and he always risked getting in trouble by taking her on the ride-on lawn mower. But it was one of her favorite activities, so he never listened to us. Cam would always tell me to give him heck for that, but I never did. I didn't want to upset him because I was always worrying about his high blood pressure. Over the years it had become quite high and even medication didn't help much. I never wanted to hurt his feelings, plus I wanted Jesse to spend as much time as possible with him. I wasn't sure how much more time they would have together.

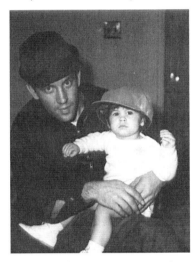 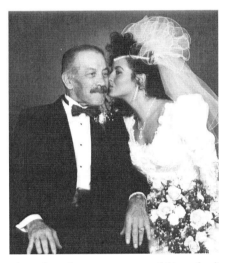

(Dad and me at One year) *(Dad and me on my wedding day)*

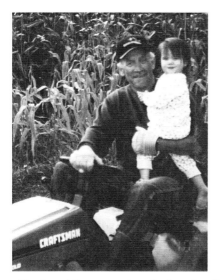 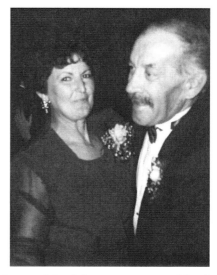

(Dad and Jesse mowing the lawn) *(Mom and Dad dancing at my wedding)*

Over the years I became very close to my brother, Steven— although I'm surprised that we didn't kill each other when growing up. I recall many altercations, some involving throwing objects. Later on, however, we developed a very strong bond. Even though he was four years younger than me, he was my protector, and I always felt safe knowing he was around.

He would do anything for me and I did the same for him. One time Steven, his girlfriend, and I went to a pub for a drink. It was really crowded and some guy thought Steven had pushed him, and all of a sudden this guy head-bonked Steven, knocked him to the ground and continued to hit him. Without a thought for the consequences, I jumped on the guy's back and wouldn't get off for anything. Steven was my little brother and I would have given my life for his. Fortunately, Steven was okay, but he did have to get a few stitches.

Steven was a very good looking guy with crystal clear blue eyes, beautiful white teeth, and a very warm, charming smile. His naturally muscular build caught the attention of many girls, and he loved every minute of it. His confidence was a force to be reckoned with. He never backed down from anyone, nor was he scared of anything. Steven had a lot of Dad in him, both the endearing qualities as well as the stubborn ones. I recall him often coming home all bruised up, either from motorbike wipe-outs or from getting into a fight.

A couple of years after graduating high school, he married his childhood sweetheart, Tammy. She was a nice girl with long curly blond hair and blue eyes. You could almost say she had a tomboy look about her, never wearing much makeup, and always motorbike riding with Steven.

Chapter 4
It All Comes Crashing Down

Now that I've given some insight into my life and the people in it, I'll continue my story and fast-forward to the events leading up to the month when this near-perfect little life of mine started to unravel, and we were plunged into one of the most difficult tests a mother and her children could be faced with.

It was May, 1998, and I was staying quite busy juggling being a wife, a mother (Jesse was three), and an entrepreneur. I had quit my sales job with a beauty supply company because Tracee and I had started up our own dating service called "Friend of a Friend Introductions." Both of us had been unhappy at our jobs, and I was tired of being on the road so much. Tracee and I had been spending so much time together, often brainstorming ideas for starting our own company. Thus "Friend of a Friend Introductions" was born.

It didn't take long for our business to become quite popular and well known. We served people from all around the Fraser River Valley and Vancouver who wanted to meet a partner for a long-term, serious relationship. Most of our clientele were divorced or widowed people who were finding it difficult to know where to meet someone compatible. Bringing lonely people together and seeing them become happy was very rewarding. Tracee and I loved it, and we were pretty good at finding great matches. Many of the people we matched went on to get married. Some even began a family.

I was really enjoying life. My marriage was great, I loved being a mother, and was filled with excitement about the arrival of our second child, scheduled to arrive around the middle of June. This pregnancy had gone very smoothly, very similar to my pregnancy with Jesse, only I had gained a few more pounds this time.

I had a lot to be thankful for. However, I was a little concerned because Jesse was showing some delays. She wasn't following the typical three-year-old development. We took her for many assessments and evaluations, but all the professionals would say is that she was totally fine, just a little late to develop in a few areas. They suggested putting her in preschool early. Still, I was worried that there was more to it. As a parent it's quite typical to compare your child with other children their age, and I was noticing all my other friends' three-year-olds were talking and doing things that Jesse wasn't. They seemed to be breezing through their milestones. Jesse had a limited vocabulary and difficulty communicating with anyone. Potty training was starting to look like an impossibility.

I began to do some of my own investigating—not to prove the professionals wrong, because in fact I wanted desperately to believe nothing was wrong with my beautiful baby girl. However, I believe a mother knows when something just isn't right. From the medical information I gathered online I realized that Jesse displayed a few symptoms of autism, a neurological disorder affecting IQ and social development. I'd never known anyone with autism, and had only *heard* of the term before, but from what I gathered some of the signs were there. For example, Jesse could recite the alphabet by memory, but couldn't put more than a couple words together. From this I knew she wasn't delayed, because no other three-year-old I knew could recite the alphabet. Autistics can be very advanced in some ways and behind in others. Yet, Jesse also displayed many characteristics which were far from autistic, especially her abundantly happy, social personality

Jesse loved the cartoon "Arthur," and had a large collection of videos that she would watch over and over. She especially loved Arthur's little sister, D.W. After watching an episode once or twice, she had memorized all of D.W.'s lines. This also could be interpreted as an autistic trait but my concerns fell on doctor's deaf ears. Granted, I was a worry wart and came by it honestly, so I wrestled with the idea that I *could* be overreacting.

I tried not to focus on Jesse's oddities, but to be honest it gnawed at me from time to time. It probably would be fair to say that sometimes I felt a little cheated. I was supposed to have this perfect child, along with the perfect husband, complete with a white picket fence. Little did I know this was going to be minor compared to what was coming my way. My world was about to completely turn upside down and inside out.

Friday, May 29, 1998, I was getting ready for work. Cam had taken Jesse to my parents' house to for them to baby-sit her when I called him saying I couldn't stand up because I was experiencing dreadful cramping coupled with a lot of pain. I didn't know what was happening and was very scared. I was three weeks from my due date, but Jesse had been three weeks early, so I thought this baby might simply be coming early too.

Cam rushed home, and seeing how much pain I was in he immediately said, "We need to go to the hospital right now." Within twenty minutes I was lying down in a hospital bed. I knew something wasn't right and was dreadfully worried about the fate of my baby.

A nurse came into my room to hook me up to a monitor, when all of a sudden I felt a huge gush of fluid soak the bed. I looked at Cam and could literally see the color leave his face. In a panic I asked him, "Did my water just break?" No words came from his lips. His frantic expression told me this was really bad.

The nurse said, "No, honey, that's blood. But don't worry. You're going to be fine. I'll be right back with the doctor."

How did she know I'd be fine? I didn't even care if I would be fine. I only cared about my baby being fine. The next few minutes were terrifying. Why was this happening? Was my baby going to be okay? I became numb to the physical pain, but emotionally I was dying.

The gynecologist came immediately and the rest was a blur. The next thing I knew, I was being wheeled into the operating room. I was told my placenta had ruptured and I needed an emergency C-section. I had lost a lot of blood and there was no time for questions.

Surgery was over in less than twenty minutes. When I became conscious I was very groggy and disoriented and it took me a few minutes to realize where I was and why I was there. A nurse standing on the other side of the room looked my way and saw I was starting to stir, so she came to my side. I was afraid to ask the question, but needed to know. "How is my baby?" I whispered.

With a forced smile she replied, "There have been some complications, honey, but he's in good hands. The doctors are working on him right now. We think he might have a heart problem."

I remembered thinking, *She said him.* That meant I had a baby boy. But before I could articulate any joy, a rush of terror filled my senses. A what? A heart problem? What did that mean? Would he have to have a heart transplant? How could this have happened without the doctors detecting it? And why did this happen? Having a baby is supposed to be one of the most beautiful experiences in one's life.

It was all too much. I screamed, "I want to see him! I need to be with him! He needs me!" I tried to jump out of my bed, but excruciating pain crippled any attempt of escape. I felt like I was being cut in half.

"As soon as he's stable you can see him," she replied, "but right now I'll go get your husband for you."

Oh my God, I thought. *Poor Cam! How is he handling all this?*

Cam came into my room and I had never seen such despair in his face before. I could tell he was trying to out up a brave front, but after six years together this was the first time I had seen this kind of intense fear in his eyes. Immediately I knew our situation was grave. He held my hand and told me how proud he was of me and how much he loved me. "We have our baby boy," he said as tears began to fill his eyes.

"Will he be okay? Have you seen him?" I asked.

Cam said he had gotten a little glimpse, but so many doctors and nurses were around him, and there were so many machines hooked up to him that he hadn't been able to see what he looked like.

Cam tried his best to assure me everything would be okay, and I'd be able to see him soon. I'm not sure where it came from, but the next words from my mouth were, "His name is going to be Avery." (Cam had wanted the name Griffin). With a gentle smile Cam replied, "Okay, Avery it is."

Soon one of the doctors came to talk to us. He explained that Avery was on life support and in critical condition. A team of doctors were on their way from Children's Hospital in Vancouver, two hours away. Avery had a very serious, life-threatening heart defect and needed to be in a more specialized hospital that would be able to help him.

I lay helpless while my world fell apart. I wanted to be anesthetized again, to go back to sleep where I didn't have to cope. I knew I was far too weak of a person to endure a crisis of this magnitude. I had barely survived the death of my beloved dog Sam. How in the world could I survive *this*?

During my surgery Cam had called my Mom and Dad, his parents, Tracee, Nikcole, Rhonda, and some of our other close friends to fill them in on what was happening. They were all waiting to see me after surgery, but I didn't really want to see anyone. By the time I was out of recovery, they had already arrived and had been told about the situation.

I was on a lot of morphine for the pain, and I wondered if the doctors and nurses also wanted to keep me semi-unconscious so I wouldn't go crazy. It didn't seem to help much except to haze my mind. Yes, it eased some of my physical pain, but no amount of morphine could have put a buffer on my deep despair.

Dad was taking all this particularly hard. He didn't know what to say, and couldn't stay in one spot. He kept walking in and out of the room. I was his baby girl, but I was hurting so bad and there was nothing he could do about it. All the years he protected me and now all he could do was look on helplessly. Everyone was in disbelief, not knowing what to say. Thank God for my Mom. I had no strength for words, but just her being there was a comfort and helped keep me from wanting a morphine overdose.

Fighting back the tears, Tracee said to me, "You have your baby boy."

I knew she was trying her best to be positive, and I could see how proud she was of me, but the words cut like a knife. Yes I had my baby boy, but for how long?

Finally after what seemed like an eternity, but probably only a few hours, the transport team had Avery stabilized enough to transport him to Children's Hospital. They brought him in to see me before they left. I felt like I was in the twilight zone as I watched the doctors push in a contraption of some sort and wheel it towards me. I noticed a tiny bundle inside, encapsulated in a clear dome riddled with machines. Those machines were breathing for him and keeping him alive. I put my hand through the only hole in the incubator and held his little hand. I couldn't see much of his face. It was covered with breathing tubes and tape. I was only able to see him for a minute. It wasn't enough, but I didn't have a choice. I probably couldn't have borne much more anyway, seeing my little baby so desperately sick and clinging to life, while I couldn't even hold him, nor let him know I was here and would never leave him if I had a choice.

There wasn't enough room for Cam in the ambulance, so Rob drove him to the hospital, and Cam's dad followed. I desperately needed to be with Avery, but I'd just had surgery, and was still hooked up to several machines. It was an impossible situation, and I wanted out. I wished I were in a coma. For the first time in my life I understood how people could feel so defeated that they no longer had the will to continue living. Thankfully and miraculously, I did just the opposite. Instead of sliding into despair, a relentless determination came over me.

I desperately tried everything to get discharged, but the doctors wouldn't do it. I was told that after my catheter was removed the next day, I could be transferred to Women's Hospital, which was a part of Children's Hospital. Tomorrow? Tomorrow was a lifetime away. I couldn't even imagine being separated from my newborn baby. It was impossible to put into words. Have you ever seen a calf being taken away from its mother? Normally cows are so passive, but I remembered one time seeing a momma cow bellow and cry in a rage when the farmer came into the field and took her baby away. Displaying no compassion, he clumsily picked up the calf, placed it in the dirty wheelbarrow, and briskly wheeled it away. The momma chased the farmer trying to knock him down by bunting his body with her head. It broke my heart, and back then I could have only imagined what she must have felt like. Now I knew; now I was that momma cow.

Cam phoned me after he got to Children's Hospital. Avery had arrived there an hour earlier. One of the doctors later described their trip: "At one point I was scared for our lives! The ambulance attendant was driving so fast as we went over Vancouver's most densely-traveled bridge on a busy Friday morning that it was like the parting of the Red Sea."

Cam told me that shortly after arrival, he had met with Avery's cardiologist, Dr. Human. For a split second I felt as though I were in another world. *What's happening? What kind of name is 'Dr. Human'? I really have been transported to the Twilight Zone. I have no control over what will happen next.* I'd never had any clue what it felt like to experience a breakdown, but I knew one must surely be headed my way.

Cam said he had instantly liked Dr. Human, and described him as a very kind and compassionate man. He had known Cam was in shock and at a complete loss in this situation. As gently as possible he had begun to discuss Avery's course of treatment, explaining to Cam that Avery was in ICU (Intensive Care Unit). His heart wasn't putting out much blood flow to the rest of his organs, and he'd likely need an emergency heart surgery called a "balloon septostomy." This would entail actually ripping a small hole in Avery's heart to provide better blood flow to the lungs.

Dr Human had explained that Avery had a fairly rare heart defect called "transposition of the great arteries" (TGA for short). His great arteries were reversed and his blood flow was going in the wrong direction. He was blue and had dangerously low oxygen saturations of 30–40%. They should have been 97–100%.

Avery was three weeks early and 5.6 pounds, so the doctors weren't certain how to proceed because they feared he wasn't strong enough to survive the open heart surgery needed to save his life. They were phoning hospitals all around North America to get advice on the safest route to take. They themselves had only treated a few cases of premature TGAs, and none of them had survived, because the TGA babies were premature and underweight and weren't strong enough to survive being on the heart and lung machine.

From their past experiences, the doctors concluded it was most important for Avery to reach a minimum of seven pounds before surgery could be done with any chance of success.

The open heart surgery Avery would ultimately need to save his life was called "the Switch." This entailed the surgeon cutting off and switching the great arteries to make Avery's heart function normally. It was quite risky because his heart was the size of a walnut, and the arteries were the size of pins. If the arteries were to kink upon switching, this would cause a heart attack. Because Avery was too small and unstable, the doctors decided the safest choice was to proceed with the balloon septostomy with the hope this would provide more time for him to get stronger.

Within hours of arriving at Children's Hospital, Avery was in the OR (Operating Room) receiving his first heart surgery. Cam, Rob, and Cam's dad waited in one of the parent's rooms while Dr. Human performed the procedure. Two hours later they received the news that all had gone well. Avery was back in ICU.

As soon as Cam had the opportunity he phoned my cell to tell me the news. Needless to say, I was relieved to hear it, but at the same time I was so far away and felt totally helpless. It was the worst feeling I had ever felt in my life. I wanted to rip my catheter out right there and hijack a car to go be with my son. It was probably a good thing I was so sedated on morphine or else I might have tried.

I talked to Cam quite a few times that day. I was trying to visualize his description of the ICU, but it was difficult to imagine a large open room filled with very sick babies and children. All the patients were on life support attached to many monitors and machines with a nurse stationed at every bedside. Other than the constant bells and whistles going off from the machines, Cam said it was calm and quiet. It was impossible to conceive that my son was one of the sick little babies hooked up to all those machines.

How will I survive this? I wondered. *More importantly, how will Avery?*

Chapter 5
The Aftermath

Saturday May 30, 1998

My journal begins with these words: Today is the longest day in my life. The ride in the transfer ambulance to Women's and Children's Hospital is long and painful. Every tiny bump feels like my stitches are being ripped out. Thank God my Mom is able to ride with me while Jesse stays home with Dad. The worst part of the ride is not knowing what to expect once it ends. Part of me can't wait to be with my newborn son, but much of me is too terrified to face him. I already love him so much. I am afraid to love him more because I don't know how I will survive the pain if I lose him.

When I arrive at my hospital room, Cam is there waiting for us. We embrace in a tight, very long hug, blending our tears in each others' cheeks. He then tells me Avery is hanging on but very unstable.

It has been only twenty-four hours since my surgery, and I can't walk any distance yet, so with Cam's help I manage to shuffle into a wheelchair. The wheelchair ride to ICU seems to take forever. I can't wait to see Avery, but I don't know what to expect. I'm in a complete fog, staring around at my surroundings, noticing all the other lost souls with helpless, vacant faces walking down the corridors of the hospital. How fast a life can be plunged into despair. No one ever prepares you for something like this … perhaps because nobody can.

I already know that my life has been changed forever, but going into ICU is a staggering experience. When Cam brings me to Avery's bedside where he lays fighting for his life, I feel the fight-or-flight instinct fill my body. I keep thinking, *I can't deal with this. I'm far too weak a person. My whole life had been lived through rose-colored glasses, so how on earth can I be equipped to handle this?*

Somehow a morsel of strength wiggles its way into my soul and I realize, *As long as Avery can stay and fight, I must too.*

Avery is encapsulated in a plastic incubator resembling a see-through dome, and is hooked up to many machines with numerous wires and tubes attached to him. With the breathing tube taped to his face, I can't see what he looks like. I'm only able to notice he has a full head of golden brown hair and perfectly-shaped little eyebrows, with long curled eyelashes.

I am his mom, yet I feel invisible. He is surrounded by many doctors and nurses trying to stabilize him. I ask one of the nurses, "Is he going to be okay?"

She says, "I really don't know. He's a very sick little baby." Her response is so cold. I wish she would have lied … or that I had never asked the question.

I feel like a deer caught in the headlights, frozen with fear. I can't hold or even touch Avery because he is so unstable and attached to so much equipment. His heart rate and oxygen saturations are continuously bouncing all over the place and the alarms on his monitors are always sounding. All I can do is pray and remind myself to breathe, but it's painfully difficult because I'm terrified he might die before I even have a chance to hold him.

I don't even know how I'm coping. I have always been such a wimp in stressful situations. Humans must have some kind of mechanism that kicks in when facing intolerable circumstances.

Not long after I arrive in ICU, Dr. Human comes to talk with us. I can see why Cam spoke so highly of him when they met yesterday. He is a handsome, meticulously well-put-together man in his mid-forties, with big brown compassionate eyes, and a charming, soothing South African accent. With warmth and empathy, he explains to us that Avery's heart condition, though very complicated, is fixable. However, Avery is so small and very unstable, the outcome is unpredictable. The next step is to wait a few days for him to get him stable enough to come off life support and breathe on his own. This process is called "extubation."

My state of mind makes it very difficult for me to remain focused on what Dr. Human tells us. I feel like a tornado has swept me up and landed me on another planet. I am full of uncontrollable tears and can't stop trembling.

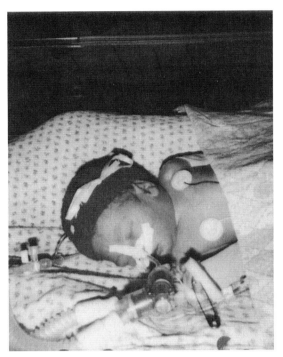

(Avery, two days old)

June 3

Today I'm not sure if I'll be able to maintain enough mental strength to continue writing in my journal, but I decide to do my best. I think it's important to have these words to reflect on in years to come. I have no idea what has compelled me to start this journal. I haven't even written in my diary for fifteen years.

A few days have gone by and Avery seems to be staying the same, induced to sleep twenty-four hours a day. The medication he is on to keep him comfortable also keeps him sleeping. Cam and I must look like zombies as we sit here all day and most of the night just staring at him and making the odd small talk with the nurses.

It's apparent the nurses are becoming very fond of Avery. They spike up his thick, beautiful, golden brown hair, and take many pictures of him with a Polaroid instant camera. Then they decorate around the picture frames with colorful nail polish, and tape them to his incubator. I can't help but wonder if these pictures are all I'm going to have one day. I try desperately not to think that way, but sometimes I just can't help it.

Our camera is at home, but I don't feel like taking any pictures anyway. People only take pictures of good things, and this situation is just the opposite. I think the nurses are taking pictures of him in case he dies. They know we'd want some pictures of him. Many parents have left this hospital with only a picture. It's not fair. I can't be one of those parents. I will do anything to ensure Avery's survival, but I'm helpless, aside from my desperate prayers and cries to God for help.

There are many doctors coming in and out of ICU, checking on Avery constantly. One doctor I have grown to like is Dr. Adderley (the head of ICU). He is an unusual-looking man, kind of Einsteinish. With his longer, messy, gray hair, and wrinkled clothes, he often looks disheveled, but he is a terrific doctor. I don't think he gets much sleep because I never see him without a coffee in his hand, whether it's 9:00 at night, or 4:00 in the morning. He literally spends hours at Avery's bedside trying to figure out how best to stabilize him enough to breathe on his own.

In the meantime, Avery is being fed only intravenously. He needs all the nutrients from breast milk to help him get bigger and stronger, so I have been pumping my milk every three hours at the hospital. How I have kept up my milk production is beyond me, especially since stress often can stop breast milk production. The nurses and doctors said that feeding a sick baby mother's milk can mean the difference between living and dying. Talk about pressure!

I already feel like I have become a pro pumper, and can even pump both breasts at the same time. It's kind of comical to think about how I must look as I pull up my knees and use them to prop up the bottles, freeing my hands so I can browse through magazines.

However, today's experience almost sends me over the edge. After I start pumping I look down, only to see that my milk has turned a bright, almost neon green. I'm horrified. My milk has gone bad! The stress has finally got to me. Somehow I manage to finish pumping then proceed to the nurses' station where mothers take their milk to be labeled before it gets sent to the freezer. I sheepishly pass it to the nurse while saying with a glowing red face, "I think...um...I think my milk has gone bad."

She takes a look at both bottles, and I'm perplexed to see a slight grin emerge on her face. She asks me, "What did you eat for dinner?"

I haven't eaten much at all, but take a moment to think before I quietly reply, "Some pasta with pesto."

I hear her chuckle under her breath before she assures me my milk is just fine, and that eating pesto or beets changes a mother's milk color. Oh boy, do I ever laugh! It feels so good to laugh. I thought I had forgotten how. I'm sure I'll be a little amused every time I open the freezer to put more milk in because I'll see this bright green "alien" milk in the freezer with my name on it, amongst all the other moms' nice cream-colored milk. I smirk as I wonder what the other moms will think, and their curiosity about "Who is this Kim Gemmell with neon green milk?"

Since we're spending so much time at Avery's bedside (close to eighteen hours a day), we're getting to know the nurses pretty well.

Some have signed up to be Avery's primary nurse. This means that whenever it's their twelve-hour shift, they'll be with Avery.

Our favorite nurse is Bonnie. She's a golfer, as is Cam, so they have a lot of golf talk going on. Bonnie is one of the smartest, most confident people I have ever met. Sometimes I think she knows more than the doctors. She's a beautiful girl in her early thirties with gorgeous long, dark curly hair. She wears these funny looking red clogs that match her full, ruby lips. I have to laugh when she says how pretty I am considering I had just had an emergency C-section. My eyes are so puffy from crying I look like a jellyfish. Plus, I'm white as a ghost from being anemic. For the first time since I can remember I could care less how I look. Just the same, I'm flattered by Bonnie's comment.

Linda is another one of Avery's primary nurses. She's probably in her mid-thirties, married, and has two young boys. It's a comfort to me when she is working with Avery. Her large brown, compassionate eyes provide warmth when she speaks to me. She knows all too well what it's like to have a very sick baby. A few years ago her youngest son, Cameron, had been born three months early. He was very sick and spent many months at Children's Hospital. Fortunately, he survived and now is a healthy young boy. She says Avery reminds her of Cameron. Linda has quickly developed a bond with Avery and even phones in on her days off to see how he's doing.

Chapter 6
A Visit From Home

June 4

Today is an exciting day because Mom and Dad are coming for their first visit to see us at Children's Hospital, and are bringing Jesse with them. I'm very anxious. It seems so long ago since I've seen Jesse's beautiful little face, yet it has only been a week. In the midst of all this heaviness it helps to have something to look forward to.

Dad phones us once they arrive in the parking lot, so Cam and I walk outside to meet them. Right away I get a glimpse of Jesse walking toward us. She's a sight for my sore eyes and looks more beautiful than ever in her favorite blue flower print dress, wearing her familiar amazing smile. When she spots me, her big blue eyes become larger than saucers. She begins to run towards me and leaps into my arms. Tears filled with both joy and sorrow stream down my face and our tight embrace lasts for minutes.

It's a joyous reunion, and I'm beginning to realize many things for the first time. I am able to see Jesse with new eyes. She is healthy, vibrant, and full of life. I can see her for the remarkable gift she is. I can't even believe I have been so distraught about her delays. How foolish of me. Here my son is lying in ICU fighting for his life, and a week ago I was stressed about potty training. My life is taking on a whole new perspective. Avery is only a few days old, but he is already teaching me some very valuable lessons.

After a little chitchat, Cam and I bring them in to see Avery. Mom and Dad are instantly so in love with him, but I can also see the fear in their eyes. I know it well; I have been looking at it every day in the mirror.

Their admiration for his strong will fills their faces. Jesse smiles when she looks at Avery, and stares at him for a long time. It's a difficult moment for all of us to take in, while we try to remain strong for each other, especially for Jesse. She's only three, and I can see she's very confused. Her limited vocabulary makes it too much of a challenge for her to ask any questions, and no amount of explaining can help her understand anything going on right now. It breaks my heart to realize that nothing in her world makes any sense anymore.

Just as heartbreaking is seeing my Dad cry. He tries to conceal his tears, but he is too overcome with emotion. I can only remember one other time I have seen him cry. I was fifteen and Dad had just buried my dog Sam in our back yard. I was devastated. Sam had been with me for fifteen years and we had grown up together. Sam walked me to school every morning, and was there to greet me and to walk me home when the bell went. Every kid in the school was friends with Sam. Many would try playing with him, but he never moved his eyes from the old school door until he saw me come out. He was my best friend in the world.

Old age caused Sam's demise. His sight was starting to fail, and he had wandered into the street where he was hit by a car. The driver left Sam to die on the side of the road. I knew that burying Sam was going to be extremely difficult for Dad, and I was starting to worry a little because he had been outside the house for a long time. When I walked outside I saw him sitting on the steps, his head buried in his hands, crying. As the tears began to fall from my own eyes, I sat down beside him and put my arm around him. Dad was sad for my loss but I think he was also sad because he couldn't do anything about it.

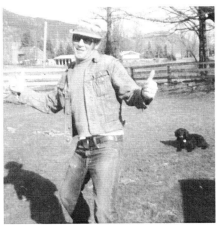

(Dad and Sam)

We had been sitting silently on the steps for a while when I reminded him of the time when he *had* been able to save Sam's life many years earlier. I was in grade four, and Dad was on his way home from work when he saw Sam lying on the side of the road. He had been hit by a car on his way to meet me after school, and had been left for dead. He fell limp into Dad's arms, and Dad laid him down on the truck seat and raced to the veterinarian. When he walked in carrying Sam in his arms he said to the vet, "I don't care if you have to make a bionic dog of him, but whatever you do, don't let him die." He then came home and with a leap of faith told me that I had nothing to worry about—Sam had been hit by a car but was going to be just fine. Fortunately he was, after a few weeks in the hospital and a huge vet bill. I knew my Dad: he would have re-mortgaged the house to ensure he could pay for Sam's survival.

Back then, it was clear to see how he would have done anything to spare me from pain. As much as he wants to, he can't do that this time.

Despite these dreadful circumstances, it's nice to see Mom, Dad, and Jesse today. I don't want them to leave. I want to bury my body in their arms and scream, "Help me! Don't leave me!"

When it's time to go, we all walk outside to say our goodbyes. Jesse doesn't want to leave us, and won't let go of me. She hugs my legs as hard as her little arms can. She's crying and yelling, "Please don't leave me, Mommy!"

It's too devastating. I feel like I'm being torn in two, but I have no choice. Avery is sick and he needs me more. Finally Dad scoops Jesse into his arms and says in his quiet, low-toned voice, "Let's go and get an ice cream cone, honey." Then he carries her away, screaming and crying all the way back to their car. It takes everything in me to not chase after them. I listen to her desperate cries until they fade into the distance.

Cam goes back inside to be with Avery, but I need some time to collect my thoughts. I don't get very far on my walk when the levy of tears burst. Everything is building up and I simply can't handle it anymore. I sit down on the ground, hang my head, and sob. When I open my eyes, surprise and wonder fill my senses: I see a four-leaf clover inches from my nose!

I remember all the four-leaf clovers I had found at my Grandma's farm, and how she couldn't believe how often I found them. Could this be a sign from Grandma? Is she trying to tell me everything is going to be okay? A sense of calm partially replaces my fear. I pluck the clover from the ground, wipe away the tears, and walk back to the hospital with hope restored.

Chapter 7
What Next?

June 5

The Today I'm discharged from Women's Hospital. I feel grateful for the six days I was able to stay there. It was so convenient because it's only a few minutes walk to ICU and Cam was able to sleep on a cot beside my bed.

Fortunately, we find a handy and inexpensive place to stay. We discover there are RVs in the back hospital parking lot. When we inquire, we find out that RV hookup is available for out of town patients for only ten dollars a day. Cam's parents, Madge and Steve, offer their motor home to us, and we gratefully accept. Steve drives it and parks it in the lot, and Madge follows him in their car. This will be our new home for the time being. Even though we'll spend ninety percent of our time in the hospital, I'm glad we'll have some privacy and a place to lay our heads for a few hours when needed.

This afternoon we receive a visit from my brother Steven and Tammy. Shortly after their arrival Tammy turns to me and says, "My mom has something important she needs to talk to you about."

I ask, "Do you know what it is?"

Tammy replies, "Well, it's something to do with an important message she has for you. And she wants to speak with you as soon as possible."

I am very curious and tell Tammy I'll phone her right away. I don't know Mrs. Johnston all that well, but from what I do know, I really like her. She is kind and generous, and has soft, friendly brown eyes. She listens intently when anyone speaks to her, and is genuinely concerned for people's welfare. Mrs. Johnston is a very spiritual person and is quite involved with her church. She knows the Bible better than anyone I know, and can recite almost any verse by memory. She has an extremely close relationship with God. I'm not as devout as her, although I have a strong faith and occasionally go to church.

I think her message might have some religious connotation, but I never expect to hear what she has to say to me. She says, "Kim, I went to my special place on our farm where I go to talk to God. Sometimes, very rarely, God will write to me through my pen. I was praying for Avery when I received a very clear message from God. He told me that Avery will have some very turbulent times, but he will come through them all and live to be strong and healthy."

My mouth nearly drops to the floor.

Wow! How does a person *begin* to respond to a statement like that? Many seconds pass before I ask, "Really? Are you sure of this?"

She replies, "I would never tell you if I wasn't certain, Kim."

In a state of shock, I thank her very much for the prayer and the message, and tell her I hope she is right. After I hang up the phone I walk aimlessly around the hospital for a while, trying to gather my thoughts. *Could this be true, or has Mrs. Johnston gone cuckoo? I want so desperately to believe her, and I know she would have never gone out on such a limb if it wasn't true. She would have never given me such blind faith, or hope. So I will cling to her words every day and pray she is right.*

… although it is unsettling what she said about the turbulent times Avery will go through.

June 6

Today starts off as an exciting day full of hope. The doctors think Avery is ready for extubation, and will be able to breathe on his own. Cam and I can't watch as the tubes are taken out. The nurses tell us it isn't a pleasant procedure and will be difficult to watch. I'm bursting with anticipation. I'll finally get to see my son's face without all the tubes and other stuff covering it. Anxiously we wait in the parents' lounge for the word. Less than ten minutes pass before Bonnie comes in with a big smile bringing good news: "Avery is extubated and breathing on his own."

I can hear him crying as we approach his bed. It is the first time I can hear his little voice. His cry sounds like a wounded lamb, but it is music to my ears. After eight long days, I am about to hold my son for the first time. My body tingles with nervous excitement when Bonnie carefully places Avery in my arms. All the machines and wires attached to his body make holding him a little awkward, but I don't care. I'm finally able to hold my baby.

Wow! As I stare at this little miracle, I see he is even more beautiful than I had imagined. It's an incredible feeling as I look down at my brave baby boy. I can't believe how much love and admiration I feel for this little guy. With his tiny body nestled in my arms, I begin to sing to him the only song I can think of, the Barney theme song: "I love you. You love me. We're a happy family…"

As I sing, Avery begins to blink then squints to open his eyes for the first time. He finally gets to see his mom. Cam says, "He probably wants to check out the awful singer who's holding him." This brings much laughter, probably because it's true. I'm the first to admit I can't carry a tune to save my life, yet it has never stopped me from belting out a song if I feel so inclined. (I did have to give up on going to Karaoke, however, because no one wanted to go with me anymore.)

Taking my first look at Avery's curious blue eyes, furiously blinking and trying to focus, is overwhelming. I think to myself, "I never want to let him go. I will die if he doesn't come through this."

Over the next few hours Cam and I take turns holding Avery. I know we still have a long road ahead of us, but for the moment I can't help but smile. It is the most joyous time I've had since hearing the nurse tell me I had delivered a baby boy.

Our contentment becomes short-lived when early evening arrives and it becomes evident that Avery is beginning to struggle with his breathing. He breaks out into a sweat, and his heart rate jumps to 196. What had started out as a great day is now spiraling downwards fast. The doctors assess him to decide what to do. They inform us, "Avery's oxygen saturations are dangerously low. His lungs are being flooded by too much blood flow, and his body is starting to shut down."

"No, no, no, this can't be happening," I cry. Bonnie gently touches my shoulder. "Dr. Adderley is calling in Dr. Jacques LeBlanc. He's the head of cardiothoracic surgery. The doctors fear Avery is heading for cardiac arrest and will need emergency heart surgery to slow down the blood flow to his lungs.

Today started out so full of hope, but now I feel like I'm in some kind of altered state too difficult to describe—kind of numb, almost mechanical. We sit quietly in a vegetative condition while we wait for the surgeon to arrive. Not knowing what is happening from one moment to the next, and feeling so useless, is too emotionally painful. Until now I haven't known the feeling of truly helpless desperation. I have been so unaware of the harsh blows life is capable of delivering.

Avery's breathing is becoming so labored that the breathing tubes must go back in. I was able to hold my son for the first time today, now I don't know when I'll be able to hold him again. I'm ready to crumble to pieces. The four-leaf clover and God's message through Mrs. Johnston are the only things keeping me sane.

At about 8:00 p.m., a handsome, stocky man, seemingly larger than life, walks in to ICU. He has thick, wavy, salt-and-pepper hair, and a trimmed beard framing his square jaw. His confident stride tells me this must be Dr. LeBlanc. He's all dressed up in a dapper, camel-colored, expensive suit. We must have disrupted him from an important affair. I think, *I hope we didn't put him in a bad mood because we threw a wrench into his important evening plans.*

With a certain self assurance he walks right up to us and introduces himself. From his accent I can tell he is French Canadian. For some reason I become extremely nervous in his presence, and probably a little intimidated. I want him to like me. I need him to save my son. Upon our introduction I blurt out, "Je parle un petite peu du Français." (I speak a little bit of French).

Did I say that out loud? Oh my God, I feel so stupid—but it just came out.

Raising an eyebrow he replies, "Your French is well spoken."

Beginning to blush, I sheepishly thank him. *Why the heck did I say that? Oh well … he has to know I'm in a state of shock.*

Bonnie had told me earlier that Dr. LeBlanc is one of the best heart surgeons in North America. Seeing him now, I'm not surprised. His confident gait and in-charge composure make his self assurance evident. Bonnie admitted she used to have a little crush on him. I can understand, I have just met him and he appears larger than life.

When he shakes my hand I can't help but notice how big his hands are. They are huge. I can't imagine them operating on Avery's little heart.

In laymen's terms he explains that newborn babies have a connection between the aorta and pulmonary artery called the "ductus arteriosus." In uteri, this connection allows oxygen-rich blood to pass through the lungs into the body because the baby receives oxygen from his mother. Once the baby is born and the umbilical cord is cut, the baby's own lungs start to work and process the oxygen the body needs. This duct is not needed anymore and therefore the opening will close naturally. Avery's opening didn't close, and his lungs are being flooded with blood. He is literally drowning in his own blood. Dr. LeBlanc's job is to surgically close the ductus to stop the overflow of blood.

Avery has survived one heart surgery already, and I can't help but wonder if he can make it through another. Cam and I have no alternative but to place our trust in Dr. LeBlanc. We sign the release papers and within minutes Avery is on the operating table. I don't even have time to phone Mom and Dad to tell them what's happening. I decide not to call, since all they will do is worry more. I decide to wait for the (hopefully) good news following surgery.

For two hours Cam and I once again wait to hear the fate of our son. The minutes go by like hours. We don't dare leave the room in case we miss anything. Words cease to exist while we pace back and forth. It's hard for me to look at Cam. His hallow, vacant expression is too difficult to set eyes on. For the last hour I feel almost unconscious, incapable of stringing a thought together. I am close to a full-blown panic attack when I hear footsteps approaching. Before Cam or I have the chance to get off our chairs, the door swiftly swings open and in walks Dr. LeBlanc.

It's probably only a few seconds, but seems like forever before he begins to speak. "Surgery went well. Avery is on his way back to ICU, and you will be able to see him shortly. He is stable, but still quite critical." He adds with a subtle grin, "There is no doubt about it: he is a fighter."

Cam shakes his hand and says, "Thank you."

As I repeat Cam's sentiments, relief forces an outbreak of tears and I give Dr. LeBlanc a grateful hug. What do you say to someone who has just saved your baby's life? Thank you or any other words can never express the gratitude I feel.

With a soft pat on the back, he tells me, "It's going to be okay."

Soon after Dr LeBlanc leaves, Bonnie comes to tell us we can go back to ICU to see Avery. She throws her arms around us and tells us she knew all along that her "Little Monkey Man" had it in him to pull through. Feeling like I'm wearing cement blocks on my feet, I tightly squeeze Cam's hand as we make our way down the hallway and through the doors to ICU. Avery is sleeping and looks peaceful. Unfortunately, his little face is mostly covered by the life support machine again, but that's okay with me because it's that machine which is keeping him alive.

Throughout most of the night we sit on our stools staring at him and counting our blessings. Avery has once again pulled through another life-threatening situation, and for now he is safe. Bonnie finally tells us we look like crap and should go to our motor home and get some sleep. Besides being a really good nurse, I love how she never whitewashes anything. I don't think I can possibly sleep, but out of pure exhaustion we fall asleep the moment our heads hit the pillow.

After a few hours we wake up the following morning at the crack of dawn. I can't get to Avery quickly enough. I'm in such a hurry I don't even brush my teeth or comb my hair.

Linda has the day shift with Avery today, and as soon as we approach she promptly informs us he's stabilizing nicely. I notice he looks so much better, and his skin doesn't seem so blue. Even with all the machines and wires attached to him he looks peaceful.

Shortly after we arrive, Dr. LeBlanc comes in dressed in sports-wear. It's a Saturday and normally his day off, but he wants to check on Avery. Today he is running a marathon for a cancer charity, and as he was running down Oak Street he made a pit stop to check on Avery. Wow! I am impressed. Usually you only see things like that in the movies. He seems pleased with the stats, but mentions that it's uncertain what we can expect throughout the day. Leaving us on a positive note he tells us that if all continues going well, Avery may be extubated in a few days. I welcome the news, even though I'm too apprehensive to get my hopes up.

For the first time in a long time I actually have a slight appetite, which is a good thing considering I have already lost my post-pregnancy weight. Nikcole comes for a visit around lunch time, and we decide to get a bite to eat at the cafeteria. Being a nice sunny spring day, we sit outside for a while enjoying the fresh spring air, trying to momentarily forget the doom and gloom that surrounds us.

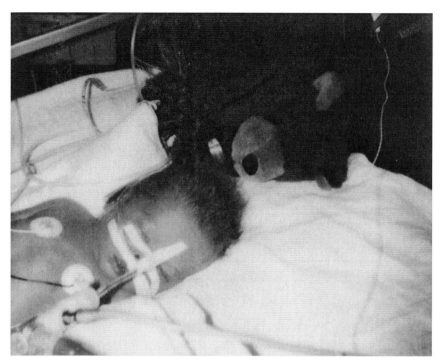

(Avery, ten days old)

Chapter 8
A Visit At Home

June 10

Avery has remained stable the past few days, and even though I feel anxious about the days ahead, my optimistic nature is slowly allowing me to embrace the thought that one day I will take him home. It's wonderful to have hope and something happy to look forward to.

It isn't until now that I'm able to lift my head slightly out of its fog to really notice our surroundings. As I mentioned before, ICU is one large room with about twenty beds, most of the time filled to capacity with sick babies and children. Only a curtain and a lot of machines separate one patient from the next. Most days the curtains are open, exposing our desperate situations to each other. I have only seen the curtains closed when a medical procedure is being performed or a baby is dying. There are a lot of parents just like us who have the same despair in their eyes.

I learn quickly that only the real sick kids stay for any length of time. The average patient spends two to three days here in ICU before they're transferred to a regular ward. We haven't had a chance to get to know many of the parents because their stays are so brief. When I see a family come and go after a day or two,

I think, *How lucky they are to be leaving so soon.* Imagine that for a minute: thinking that a parent with a child in ICU is lucky. Though most patients stays here are brief, we've had the opportunity to meet a few long-termers like ourselves.

One young woman, Amanda, who doesn't look much over twenty, has a baby here named Noah with a similar heart defect as Avery. She is from Kelowna, a town about a six-hour drive away, and other than Noah, she is here all by herself. Noah's father had left her shortly after she got pregnant. Amanda's mother has stayed in Kelowna to take care of Amanda's other child, a two year-old daughter. Amanda looks so broken and sad, so we try to talk to her and keep her company as much as possible. Mostly she sits alone all day beside Noah's bed, her long, knotted, reddish-brown hair covering most of her pale face. She often has a book or magazine in her hand, but her glazed-over, sunken eyes tell me she isn't reading much. At least Cam and I have each other; I couldn't bear to struggle through this alone.

Across the room from Avery's bed is a young Italian family, Marina and Paulo. Their three-year-old son, Anthony, had fallen into their pool and drowned. He had been under water for quite a few minutes before he was found. The doctors told them he was brain dead and there was nothing more they could do. They suggested taking him off life support and letting him go peacefully. The family can't accept that, and aren't ready to attempt extubation. Anthony has a perfect little round face with long, thick, curly blond hair. He looks so content and peaceful that it's hard to believe that it's only the machines keeping him alive. It's all too much to take in. Right now I'm living my worst nightmare, but I can't help but feel lucky I'm not in their shoes. At least we have hope—although I'm sure they have hope too. After all, miracles do happen.

Tina Parchi is the name of the newborn occupying the space to our left. Her parents, Ben and Lisa, are a friendly Jewish couple, both successful lawyers in their early forties and living in a very affluent part of Vancouver. Tina, their fourth child, born a few days before Avery, has a severe life-threatening abdominal infection. In addition, the family just found out Tina has cystic fibrosis. From looking at her beautiful face it's difficult to comprehend how sick she really is. Her curly, fire-engine-red hair frames her healthy, milky-white complexion. Yet looking at her mid-section, you know something is terribly wrong; her stomach is twice the size of her body, the size of a large beach ball. The surgeons have performed surgery to remove the infection, and now big sutures resembling shower curtain rings are holding her stomach together. As with so many things here, it's beyond my comprehension how difficult it must be for Lisa and Ben to see their newborn baby daughter in this way.

There is nothing sadder than the look on a parent's face whose child is in such jeopardy. It is the most anguished suffering look a person could witness. You know what I mean if you've seen it, or have experienced it yourself. Probably the best way to describe it is to say that their face looks like every ounce of blood was sucked out of them, and their bodies are limp and stooped. I notice some parents look totally defeated, while others have a flicker of hope remaining in their eyes. We talk to some of the families every once in a while and provide updates on how our babies are doing.

I wonder if Cam and I look as disheveled as most of the parents do—hair all messed up, clothes wrinkled, and our faces wearing a permanent look of despair. Once in a while we see a parent smile for a split second when a nurse says something funny to try to lift their spirits. Smiles are hard to come by, since tragedy and despair are all around us. All that surrounds us are very sick babies and young children fighting for their lives, every breath provided by a machine.

In the mist of such turmoil it has been easy to forget about the life we recently left behind. Cam and I are very fortunate to have been able to take the time off work and be at Avery's bedside day and night. Tracee is running our business with the help of our new employee, Nordina. Cam is able to take a leave of absence from his job, but unfortunately, is only able to receive the remainder of his holiday pay, amounting to around $1,500. We don't have much savings and what we do have will run out quickly. Our mortgage and car payments will eat it up in no time.

Cam's parents, and my parents as well, have told us not to worry about money, that they'll help us out financially if need be. We're thankful for their generous offers because it's one less worry. The way I feel now, I wouldn't care if my home slid into the river that lies behind it. The material things I have placed so much value on now mean nothing. I've heard this sometimes happens when you're faced with tragedy, and now I'm experiencing it firsthand. I would give up any possession I ever owned to have a healthy son. I'm certain anyone would.

I wonder how many people think about or truly appreciate the health of their children? I have been so stressed about Jesse's delays that I didn't think about the wealth of gratitude one should feel for having a healthy, happy child. I will never, never make that mistake again. I suppose it's somewhat typical for people to take things for granted, especially when life is going smoothly. It reminds me of my Grandma's leg. She never thought to truly appreciate it, or all the things it did for her, until it was gone. After that she appreciated every little good morsel life had to offer. I have always known this, but haven't given it a whole lot of thought until now.

My crash course in life appreciation is in full swing, and as a result I'm missing Jesse more than ever. Cam suggests I take a trip home and spend a day with her. Bonnie, our nurse today, thinks it's a good idea as well. Avery is still stable and the doctors feel he's recovering remarkably well—so well, in fact, that the plan is to go ahead with extubation in the next couple days.

Bonnie and Cam are right: this is probably the best time for a visit with Jesse. I can go for a day and be back in time for Avery's extubation. However, I'm reluctant and keep changing my mind even though I know Avery is in the best hands possible. I keep thinking, *But what if something goes wrong and I'm two hours away?* Avery's history this far hasn't given me much reason to believe he'll be okay while I'm gone. On the other hand, I also know Jesse needs me too. She has no clue why we had to leave her, and needs my support more than ever. After much deliberation and coaxing from Bonnie and Cam, I decide to go be with Jesse.

It's a long drive back to Chilliwack. I have difficulty seeing the road at times through all the tears that surface without warning. When I finally arrive in town, I stop at home because I have to go to the bathroom so bad I know I won't make it to Mom's. When I phone Mom she says Jesse is having her morning nap. I'm exhausted and need a nap myself, so I ask her if she would mind bringing Jesse to our house when she wakes up. For some reason I want Jesse to be with me at home. I guess I want her to know this is still our home. Plus, I need a bit of time to pull myself together. I want Jesse to see a semi-normal mom, not one who looks like she spent the last two hours crying.

Walking into our house for the first time since Avery was born feels strange. It has only been a couple weeks but it seems much longer. My comfy, cozy house, full of bright warm colors, now seems empty and cold. It's really puzzling, and appears almost as though the house has physically changed even though it's in the exact same condition as the day we left it. While I sit here all by myself, waiting for Jesse to come home, I imagine what the house would feel like with us all here as a family.

At this moment, I make a promise to God: if Avery makes it through this ordeal I'll be the happiest Mom in the world, never taking anything for granted ever again. I have made promises to myself before that fell by the wayside, but this time I know it will hold true. It's just one of those things you know. I can't explain it, but I also know that if Avery *doesn't* make it, I'll never recover. The second thought really scares me because I know I need to be here for Jesse.

I am unloading the dirty clothes we had been living in when I hear the truck pull into our driveway. I jump up and run to open the door, almost taking it off its hinges. Jesse's vibrant, enthusiastic smile tells me she's just as excited as me. We run to each other and embrace in a long, tight hug.

"Daddy? Avery?" she asks, shrugging her shoulders and pointing to the house.

I do my best to explain that Avery is still sick and won't be coming home for a while, and Daddy needs to stay with him today. I'm not sure how much she understands but it appears to satisfy her for the time being. I think she's just happy to be home, spending some time with one of us.

Mom comes up and gives me a big hug too. Now that she can see me in person I notice her studying my face and shrinking frame, while she asks how things are going. We sit and chat for a few minutes, and I get the impression she's a little surprised and perhaps proud of how I'm holding together. With tears in her eyes and a lump in her throat, she tells me she'll leave Jesse and me alone to have a nice visit.

Jesse anxiously grabs my hand and leads me into the backyard to her favorite spot, the swing set. I haven't appreciated how beautiful our back yard is until now—spacious and surrounded by huge maple and willow trees. The view of open fields and a gorgeous mountain feels therapeutic. It must feel good for Jesse as well because this is the first time she has been home since the morning Avery was born. It's wonderful to see her bursting at the seams with the excitement of being back.

We make the best out of the beautiful sunny day and play outside for a few hours. Sometimes I get so lost in watching Jesse play and chase dragonflies, I momentarily forget the tragic turn our life has taken. At one point, sitting on the grass watching Jesse play in the sandbox, I imagine what it might be like if Avery is here with us. It's a glorious moment until the threat of him *not* coming home begins to overwhelm me. I feel the tears begin to fill my eyes. This is supposed to be a happy visit, and I don't want Jesse to see me cry. I know if I get up to go inside she will follow me, so I stay where I am at, put my head down and sob.

I think I must be seeing things when, in the midst of my tears and blurry vision, I find myself again staring down upon a four-leaf clover! The only two occasions I have been on the grass since Avery was born, I have found four-leaf clovers – or maybe they found me? It must be a sign from my Grandma. I am almost sure of it now. Out of all the places to sit in our big back yard, how could it be just a coincidence that I sit down in front of a four-leaf clover? I stretch my neck and gaze into the sky. This is my Grandma's way of telling me everything is going to be okay.

"Thank you, Grandma," I say out loud. If anyone possesses the power to influence the outcome of this ordeal, I reason, it's her—next to God, of course.

As evening approaches I cook Jesse's favorite supper—chicken nuggets with macaroni—and some veggies with dip. It feels good to do something normal for a change. After supper Mom and Dad come over for a visit. Mom is getting really good at trying to stay upbeat about everything, but it has become more difficult for Dad. He has been much more quiet than usual, and even though he is trying his best to stay positive, he just isn't a good actor. Even Jesse's quirky little dance performances barely get more than a chuckle from him.

Shortly after Mom and Dad leave, the phone rings. The sound sends shockwaves through my body and I jump from my seat. I know it must be Cam, but why is he calling? I want to believe it's good news, but I'm afraid of the alternative. Quickly I pick up the phone and my trembling voice stutters, "H-h-hello." Yes, it is Cam and fortunately he has good news: Avery remains stable and is doing just fine. The news helps me to relax and enjoy the rest of the evening even more. I look forward to doing nothing but spending the evening cuddling with Jesse. I know it might be a long time before we get to spend another day together so I want to make the most of it.

We're both so exhausted from the day that we fall asleep holding each other on the couch while watching Barney videos on TV.

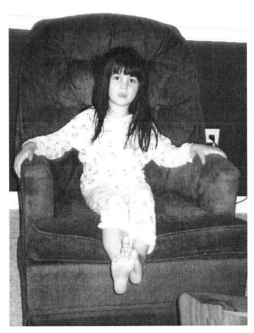

(Jesse, three years old)

June 15

Coming home to visit Jesse is a very gratifying experience, but all too soon morning comes, and the reality of returning to Vancouver sets in. While I drive Jesse back to Mom and Dad's after breakfast I tell her I must return to the hospital to be with Avery. I'm in agony as she continues to repeat, "Me come too." It breaks my heart because no matter how I hard I try, I can't get her to understand that ICU is no place for a healthy child, but at three, Jesse doesn't understand reasoning. She just wants to be with her family, and I don't blame her.

When we arrive at Mom and Dad's, Mom is outside working in the garden and Dad has gone to work. I can already feel the tears well up in my eyes as I pull in the driveway. I put my sunglasses on so no one will see me cry. When I carry Jesse out of the car and bring her to Mom, she asks how our visit was. I tell her it has been the best therapy. I think she can tell I am antsy to return to Avery, so after a few words we hug and say our good-byes.

Once again, Jesse won't let me go. Clinging to my legs she says, "Just stay, Mommy! Stay more longer!"

I notice Mom starting to tear up then she says to Jesse, "Let's go pick some flowers for Grandpa."

The distraction works, so I take the opportunity to turn and walk away. When I get into my car and speed off, it's difficult to see through the tears that blur my vision. I feel horrible to leave, like a monster, but what other choice is there? I don't want to leave Jesse, but I can hardly wait till I see Avery. It is an impossible situation. I've often heard the cliché, "God only gives you what you can handle." Well, I said many prayers on the way back to Vancouver, mostly saying that I need His help because I don't think I can handle much more.

Chapter 9
Renewed Hope

Even after doing it a hundred times, I never get used to walking through these ICU doors. My heart plummets as I push the big red button, say my name then wait for the doors to open. I feel my body turn to jelly as I walk around the corner toward Avery's bed. I start to do a fist-clenching nervous reaction as I approach the bedside. However, I feel immediate relief when I see Bonnie and Cam chatting peacefully. I know that the expressions on their faces will tell me if Avery is doing well or not. I've always been a face studier, and now I have become pretty good at it.

Cam gives me a big hug and says my visit must have been good because I look a whole lot better than when I left. After giving me a welcoming hug, Bonnie mentions that the plan is to go ahead and extubate Avery tomorrow. For the rest of the day I sit in the rocking chair holding him and singing to him. He looks so serene and content, but I can't help but wonder if he is ready this time.

June 16

The dawn is just breaking as we make our walk from the motor home to the hospital where we learn that Avery is indeed being extubated today. Bonnie is working the last of her four-day shifts, and looking forward to being part of the excitement. I can't wait to see Avery's face again without all of the tubes attached.

Cam and I get a coffee then wait in the parents' lounge while the tubes come out. We haven't finished our coffees yet when Dr. Adderley arrives with good news: Avery is breathing on his own. I can hear his cry as we approach his bed. It's the second time to hear his little voice, only this time it sounds louder and stronger than the first time. I hope this means more chance of success this time. It only took three hours after the last extubation attempt before Avery started struggling to breathe. Afternoon approaches, and Avery is still going strong, but for many hours to come we will wait every passing minute with bated breath.

Cam's parents are having their turn to look after Jesse, so Mom and Dad take the opportunity to come for a visit this afternoon. They're able to hold Avery for the first time. I can tell they are nervous at first, but after a few minutes they look content holding him. As well, today is the first time they've been able to see Avery without the tubes and tape covering his face. I can tell they're in total awe of this little person who has so much determination to live. Watching them smile makes me feel good. I want to believe this is the beginning of many good days ahead, but I'm still too scared to even think that far in the future. With two heart surgeries still to come, Avery still has a long journey ahead.

Saying goodbye to Mom and Dad is difficult, although each time is getting a little easier. I'm not sure if that's because Avery is doing better, or we're just getting used to all this upheaval. It's really surprising how we can learn to cope when tragedy strikes. I know I've said it already, but until now I really didn't believe I was capable of dealing with a situation like this.

Evening approaches and thankfully Avery has given us no surprises. Finally, about 1:00 a.m., Linda, who often works with Avery on the night shift, convinces us to go get some sleep.

About 4:00 in the morning Cam's cell phone rings. I know it can only mean something is terribly wrong. One of my biggest fears has always been that our cell phone would ring in the middle of the night and that it would be ICU. The phone is beside me but I can't answer it, so I pass it to Cam. He answers, and whispers to me that it's Linda. The conversation is short. All I hear Cam say is, "Oh no! We'll be right there!"

I panic, thinking the worst, and fall into a scrunched-up ball on the floor. I cover my ears because I don't want to hear what Cam is about to say. With panic in his voice he blurts out, "Avery's in distress and having trouble breathing! Linda said his blood oxygen saturations have dropped dramatically. Dr. Human has been called from home, and is on his way. She thinks Avery may need another emergency surgery. We need to come down now."

I can't move, I can't speak, but Cam keeps yelling in a panic, "Come on, Kim! Let's go! We've got to go now!"

I had previously thought it was just an expression, but I have become literally paralyzed with fear. My body shuts down physically and mentally and I literally can't move. Cam seems to understand and says, "It's okay. Just stay here and I'll phone you as soon as I know anything."

This is it. I'm having a breakdown and will be committed. I guess I'm not strong enough after all ... but I did give it my best.

For a few minutes I lay in a ball, and then suddenly I receive a strong urge to phone Mrs. Johnston. My fingers are shaking so much I can't dial the number properly. Finally after several attempts, I'm able to get through. It rings many times, and I'm about to hang up and try again when, thank God, she answers. I manage to stutter, "A-Avery … isn't d-doing … well."

Immediately she says, "Let's pray."

I know with Call Alert on my phone I won't miss Cam's call, so we pray together for about twenty minutes. We pray for Avery's strength to prevail and the doctors to have the knowledge to know what to do. We pray for God to provide me the strength to continue this fight. At the end of our conversation Mrs. Johnston reminds me about the message she received from God which said that Avery will go through some very rough times, but he *will* make it.

Praying with Mrs. Johnston provides a little solace, but after I hang up I think, *Why haven't I heard from Cam yet?* I can't wait any longer. I have to see Avery. It's a rainy, windy, miserable night, and I'm soaked after one minute of running through the parking lot. I'm a few feet from the hospital entrance when my cell rings. I fumble through my pocket to find it.

It's Cam. He says, "Avery is doing better. After Dr. Human arrived, he increased Avery's Digoxin medication, and it immediately improved his saturations."

Relief is an understatement as to how I feel at this moment. I reply, "Thank God! I'm almost there." I literally run through the empty halls to Avery's side. He is sleeping, breathing on his own, with his heart beating calmly. Dr. Human is still here keeping a close eye on his stats. He explains that Digoxin was the boost that Avery needs to give him more endurance so that he can continue breathing on his own. He anticipates Avery won't have to go back on life support. Dr. Human also adds, "If Avery stays stable for the next week, you might be able to take him home for a few weeks until his next surgery. I don't want to get your hopes up, but I believe there is a good chance he'll be okay to breathe on his own now."

Did he really say that? I have pushed away the thought of bringing Avery home anytime soon. Of course I'd love to bring him home, but the thought also makes me very nervous. We're two hours away from Children's Hospital, and surely our tiny local hospital won't be much assistance. I ask Dr. Human if he can come home with us. I think this is the first time I've seen him laugh. In his eloquent South African accent he replies, "Do not worry, Kim. We will make sure it is perfectly safe for you to take Avery home, and that you feel comfortable enough to do so. I promise you that."

Avery has weathered another storm, and apparently so have I. The power of prayer is amazing.

June 19

A few days pass, and it appears Dr. Human's prediction is right. Avery is doing fabulous. Slowly he's being weaned from all the monitors and medicines and so far tolerating it very well. Our spirits are high, but I'm still apprehensive about the thought of taking him home.

Nikcole comes for a visit today and brings Jesse with her. She had picked up Jesse from Mom and Dad's to spend the weekend at her house. Her daughter, Macky (Mackenzie), is a year younger than Jesse. Nikcole thought it would be nice for Jesse to have a friend to visit with. Thank God for friends like Nikcole! She's the kind of friend that people need at times like this. On average, she comes at least once a week for a visit. Something about her presence is very comforting, but I can't explain why. Sometimes she stays for hours, just hanging out with us at Avery's bedside. She gets a kick out of Bonnie, and loves her positive attitude. She admires her great sense of humor despite the trauma of working in ICU full of very sick babies and kids.

It's beyond wonderful to see Jesse again. When we bring her to see Avery she is thrilled. I wonder if she thinks this is Avery's home. I shudder to think she feels we have abandoned her—yet I can't help but think she might be feeling that way. She's old enough to know something is wrong, but not old enough to understand any kind of explanation. I keep telling her we'll all be home together as a family again but she doesn't understand. I want her to know I will never abandon her, but I don't know how to say it in a way she can comprehend. All I can do is give her lots of love whenever I get the chance. At least it's a little easier for her to leave us today because she's looking forward to her sleepover with Macky, but my heart still aches as we say goodbye.

I have been phoning Mom and Dad every day. Often, when I call, I break down and cry when hearing their voices and it takes a minute or more before I can compose myself enough to speak. It must be horrible for them to know their little girl is in so much pain. Now it's much more pleasurable to call them since Avery is doing well. They are ecstatic at the news that Avery will probably be coming home for a short stay before his next surgery.

Even though Avery is doing better, it's often difficult to be in good spirits when all I see when I look around is the sick babies and heartbroken parents. Tina is not doing any better, and Ben and Lisa have been told that her condition is bleak. The doctors can't seem to find the source of her infection, and her condition is deteriorating. They have her attached to a machine that is filtering and cleaning her blood, but it doesn't seem to be working. Ben and Lisa are starting to look very tired and drained, but they aren't giving up hope. I don't think any parent I have seen here ever completely gives up hope. For many of us, it's all we have.

Noah doesn't seem to be improving much either. He's too weak to undergo the heart surgery he needs, and apparently his defect is more complicated than the doctors had originally thought. His mom looks defeated and is having a hard time staying positive. We try to spend as much time with her as possible but she mostly just wants to be alone. I know what that feels like. Sometimes I just don't have the energy or desire to speak to anyone.

Today Anthony's one-and-a-half year old brother comes for a visit to see him for the first time since he fell in the pool. Marina and Paulo still refuse to take off his life support, even though the doctors said his scans show there is no brain activity, and he'll likely die shortly after life support has been removed. If he does live he'll be brain dead. However, they aren't ready to let go. Who could be?

Anthony's brother looks just like him, only smaller. I watch as he climbs up onto Anthony's bed, kneels beside him, while gently nudging his shoulder with his hand. Repeatedly he says, "Wake up, Anthony. Wake up." Everyone in sight begins sobbing uncontrollably. It's too much to bear, and I have to turn away. Nothing in my world makes sense anymore. Things like this should never happen to beautiful, innocent children just beginning their lives.

A little boy, about three, comes into ICU today. From the healed scar on his chest, I know he's had heart surgery at one time. I meet his father, Gord, in the lineup to get a coffee, and we start talking about what brought our children here. It turns out his son, Taylor, has the same heart defect as Avery, and had his surgery a little over three years ago. He'd been doing great and had returned to the hospital for a fairly simple procedure—a stint—that would open up an artery that had started closing. I'm not sure exactly what happened, but surgery didn't go well and he ended up on life support in ICU.

I find myself often staring at him because he is so darn cute. His long, layered blond hair frames his little face. I like to watch him when he sleeps because he looks so peaceful. When he's awake, his large, blue eyes look sad and scared, and it makes me want to cry. It's too difficult to understand why any child has to be here. He's supposed to be enjoying the summer, having a ton of fun playing outside. He's not supposed to be laying in a bed in ICU. I had known such misgivings existed; I'd just never witnessed the feelings of devastation they brought, until now.

There are more tragic stories about other families we've met during our stay but there would be far too many pages in this book if I wrote about all of them. There is too much suffering and sorrow. I can certainly see how people appreciate the joys of life much more after enduring great hardships. In the midst of these tragedies some things have begun making sense, like how my Grandma was always so happy and grateful despite losing one of her legs. She felt blessed just to be alive.

June 22

Avery has been extubated for a week and the doctors feel he's well enough to move out of ICU and go upstairs to the Observation Ward. There, however, instead of one-on-one care, there are only two nurses for every six to eight babies. The only devices he'll be attached to are a heart monitor and a machine for measuring oxygen saturation levels. This is a huge step up for us. It means we'll be able to take more responsibility for the care of Avery. Up until now, we haven't even been able to change his diaper. We're now entering the preparation phase in order to be discharged, and the thought of it is a little daunting.

Now that Avery is out of ICU, I'm able to sleep beside him in a cot. Cam sleeps in the children's playroom, which doubles as a dorm in the evening. Cots come out at night for any parents of patients who wish to sleep at the hospital. I don't want Cam to sleep in the motor home. I need the comfort of knowing he's only a few doors away.

Avery continues to do amazingly well. He's awake much more and becoming more alert to his surroundings. He also loves to be held all the time, usually only crying when Cam and I put him down. When Steven and Tammy came for a visit the other day, they could hardly believe it was Avery in the crib. They were pleasantly surprised by how much healthier and full of life he looked. They said we are looking much better as well.

June 28

I am filled with delight as we make plans to leave tomorrow. The doctors are confident Avery is ready for us to take home, and are especially pleased that he has the strength to nurse. Since extubation, and up until now, he has been getting my breast milk from an NG tube. (This was a long skinny tube inserted through his nose and extending to his stomach. Milk was poured in the tube through a funnel.) Finally, I don't have to pump my milk from the cow-like Hoover milking machine anymore. I'm not going to miss going to the mother's room every three hours. I just hope my breasts recover.

Avery will be a month old tomorrow. Even in my worst nightmares I never imagined this was how I'd be spending the first month with my new baby. I had loved the newborn stage with Jesse, and had been looking forward to doing it all over again with Avery. That was not to be, and now my only hope is Avery will make it home at all.

The plan is to stay home for about a month to give Avery time to get bigger and stronger. He needs to be at least seven pounds before his next surgery, and right now he is still his birth weight of 5.6 pounds. At one point Avery was down to 4.6 pounds, so the fact that he is back up to his birth weight pleases Dr. Human. He says that Avery needs all the love and support possible to ensure the success of his next surgery. I guarantee him it won't be a problem. He grins and says, "Oh, I know."

Then Dr. Human explains that Avery's third surgery will prepare his heart for the final open heart surgery. If Avery was to have his open heart surgery now (switching his great arteries) his heart wouldn't be able to take the drastic change in direction of his blood flow, and he'd likely suffer a heart attack. Therefore, the third surgery—a pulmonary artery band and a BT shunt—will slow down and redirect the blood flow in order to prepare his heart for the big switch. To me it all sounds Greek, but it's easy for me to trust whatever Dr. Human says. He has brought Avery this far, and I put my faith in him that he'll get him the rest of the way.

Chapter 10
Avery's Visit Home

June 29

For the first time, Avery is going to experience life outside the hospital. When I walk out the doors with him in my arms it feels almost too good to be true. Avery has never experienced the sun, and at first he squints then smiles the biggest smile I have seen yet. The warmth of the sun on his face must feel so good to him. Avery doesn't seem to mind the car ride home, and sleeps for most of the two-hour journey. Even though I'm nervous, I'm thankful for this temporary reprieve. I know it's only for a short time, but I feel blessed to have this opportunity before the next surgeries.

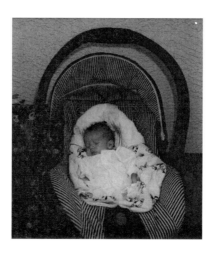

(Avery's first day in the outside world)

All our family and friends want to give us some time at home to adjust, so only Mom, Dad, Jesse, and Cam's parents are waiting for us when we get there. They hear us drive in and run to the door, and their faces light up like Christmas lights. Jesse is jumping up and down, screaming.

Avery seems undaunted by all the fuss, and for the most part enjoys being held by everyone. It's a beautiful sunny afternoon as we sit outside visiting, trying to catch up on what has been happening in Chilliwack. I never knew having just a normal day could feel so wonderful. Until now, I never thought a normal day was worth relishing.

The hours fly by and before we know it, early evening has come, so we order some takeout for dinner. There haven't been many days recently that I've been hungry for food. Up until now I mostly ate in order to keep my milk production up, and I'm getting pretty slim.

After dinner, we sit around the patio laughing and talking, just like a typical family. Avery is happy and looks so healthy that there are moments I forget about the scary road that lies ahead.

Everything on this remarkable day is intensified. My senses are heightened. Even the colors of sunset appear richer than I have ever seen before, and I feel the gratefulness my Grandma lived her life by.

By 9:00 p.m. we're all so exhausted we can barely keep our eyes open, but I don't want the evening to end. Before Mom and Dad leave, Dad comes up to me, gives me a big hug and says, "I'm so proud of you, baby." He has told me this many times throughout my life, but this time there is a much deeper sincerity in his tone.

I smile and reply, "Thanks Dad. I learned from the best." He wipes a tear from his eye.

July 6

As each day goes by, Cam and I get more comfortable having Avery at home. The house is always full of visitors. It's wonderful to see our friends and family outside the hospital. In the past, I had been used to seeing Tracee every day, and I never realized how much I had missed her until I started seeing her more often again. She has been so busy with the business that it has left her few opportunities to visit us in Vancouver. Thank goodness that Tracee was able to run things. She hadn't wanted me to even think about work, and I don't think I could have if I'd tried.

It takes at least a week of being at home before we're able get a good night's sleep, because Avery is sleeping with us. It's more comforting knowing he's beside us, but both Cam and I have been constantly waking up and checking him to make sure that he's still breathing. However, with each passing day we begin to relax a little more and learn to enjoy this opportunity to have him home with us.

A friendly health nurse has been coming over every second day to check on Avery and weigh him. I always look forward to her visits because it provides some peace of mind. She didn't recognize me at first, but I recognized her right away. She had joined Friend of a Friend many months ago. She probably hadn't recognized me at first because she'd been used to seeing me all dressed up, with hair and makeup meticulously maintained.

We've even had a few visits from Bonnie. Do I ever look forward to seeing her! It's like we have our own personal nurse. She always brings along her stethoscope and other equipment to give Avery a thorough checkup.

The best part of being home is spending time with Jesse and seeing her interact with Avery. She wants to hold him all the time, and keeps staring at him adoringly. In her world everything is okay again. She doesn't realize that we'll be leaving her again, and I try not to think about that. I often find myself repeating Grandma's words: "Appreciate every day, one day at a time." For the most part this is what I'm doing, or at least trying to do. We spend a lot of time going on walks, and hanging out at Mom and Dad's house.

We're getting nicely settled into our very welcome "normal" lifestyle, but the time is passing quickly. My dream of bringing Avery home has come true, even if just for a little while. It's so weird: I know we must return to the hospital, and yet, for the most part, I'm able to live in the moment. It's a whole new experience for me. Who would have ever thought I could enjoy cooking and even cleaning the house?

Just when I'm finding some balance and peace in my life, I'm shocked by a devastating loss.

Chapter 11
My Biggest Loss

July 18

It is Saturday morning July 18, about 10:00 a.m. when I phone Mom and Dad, like I usually do every morning. When Dad answers he sounds sleepy, which is odd because he's always been an early bird. I ask him if he'd been sleeping and he says, "No honey, I just got back from the barn and laid down to watch the horse race on TV." I ask him where Mom is and he says, "She's garage-saleing with Penni and Eileen." I tell him that Avery, Jesse, and I will be coming over to see them later that day. He says that will be great, and he'll get Mom to call me when she gets home.

I don't think about it until later, but Mom never called me back. She never got the message. It was the last conversation I would ever have with my father. I can't even remember if I told him I loved him as I often did at the end of our phone conversations. I keep going back to our phone call, but I just can't remember. It doesn't matter. He knew that I loved him more than anything.

This afternoon there's a knock on our door. I'm nursing Avery on the couch so Cam answers. There stand Mom, Penni, and Eileen, all looking immensely somber. Mom walks into the family room with a look on her face I've only seen once before. I instantly know something terrible has happened. Then it hits me like a ton of bricks. I somehow know my Dad has died. Before any words came from her mouth I ask, "Did something happen to Dad?" Her eyes fill with tears. All she can do is nod her head.

My body feels like it has fallen into a volcano as raging fire courses through my veins. I want to cover my ears to block her next words, but I know I must ask, "Did he die, Mom?"

She embraces me tightly and with a deep sigh whispers, "Yes, honey … he passed away."

No! There is no way this is really happening! I just talked to him this morning. We were coming over to visit him. I drop to the floor in the most painful despair imaginable. Mom falls to her knees facing me and pulls me into her arms. I bury my head in her chest and sob uncontrollably. The pain in my heart takes my breath away. I want to die too. I can't absorb the idea that my dad is gone. How could this possibly be happening now? We already have more than we can handle.

When I am finally able to process a thought, all I can think about is Jesse. *How will Jesse take this? In her three short years she's had way too much to bear. Her best friend in the whole world has just been taken away from her, and she won't know why. One of the only constant people in her life, who has been by her side throughout this crisis, is now gone forever.*

Things had just started to look up, and now this! Nothing makes any sense. I am so mad at God. How could this happen in the middle of our current devastation? I want to scream at God, to call Him names … but I don't. He's my biggest ally and I must not turn on Him now. I need Him to give us strength and help guide Avery and the doctors through the next surgeries.

Plus, I know that God had been trying to prepare me for this day. For some time now, I haven't been able to shake off these sporadic, unsettling feelings that Dad wasn't going to be with us much longer. They started more than a year ago. I had told Cam about my fear and he thought I was being silly and paranoid. I wanted to believe him, and would try to push those thoughts aside. I remember phoning Mom from Children's Hospital telling her to make a doctor's appointment for Dad because I was worried about his heart. She said I had enough to worry about with Avery, and Dad had just said he was feeling really good. However, I became insistent that she make an appointment, so she agreed she would. A week or so later when I asked her about it, she told me everything had checked out fine.

But my uneasy feelings *had* been a premonition from God.

Following bursts of tears and stretches of silence, slowly, painfully, Mom explains that she had come home from garage-saleing, walked into the bedroom, and found Dad on the floor. He'd had a massive heart attack while he was taking a nap. His high blood pressure had finally taken its toll. The doctors said he would've suffered no pain because it happened so fast. I hope so, but I can't be sure because Mom found Dad on the floor. I think he may have fallen out of the bed while trying to reach the phone on the bedside table.

Mom says she hasn't been able to get ahold of Steven. He and Tammy were riding their motorbikes out at the river, so she left a message for Steven to come to my house. Steven and Dad were very close. He had so much love and respect for Dad, and always wanted to be just like him. I wish so much that I could go back in time and erase this horrible day, if only to spare my brother the pain. I know he will be devastated.

A few hours after Mom left the message for Steven, we see him and Tammy come up our driveway. Mom says she doesn't know how she will be able to tell him. I can't let her go through it twice. I tell her that I'll tell him. Mom doesn't want me to, but I insist. When Steven comes to the door, he looks worried. I know he thinks something has gone wrong with Avery. The first thing he asks when he comes to the door is, "Is Avery okay?"

I say, "Yes, but something else terrible has happened."

"What?"

I hug him tightly and tell him Dad is gone. I will never forget the look on his face as he keeps repeating, "No, not our Dad. No, not our Dad." He says it at least fifteen times. I just keep holding him and saying that it isn't fair.

Mom comes into the entrance and Steven says, "Mom, tell me it isn't true."

Mom can only hug him. She says, "I only wish I could tell you it isn't true. I would give anything to tell you it isn't true."

Mom has lost the love of her life, her first and only love. She came home and found her husband of forty years dead, yet she's being so strong. I know she's trying to be strong for us, like she's always done since we were kids. Now it's my time to be strong for her. I desperately want to cushion her pain. She was at my Grandma's house when she suffered her fatal heart attack, and tried to resuscitate her. Now her husband is dead from the same cause. All this topped with the fact that her grandson has a life-threatening heart condition and needs open heart surgery. How will she able to hold it together?

I can't believe Dad is gone and won't have the chance to know his grandson. He died knowing that Avery's biggest challenges lay ahead of him. Maybe this was all too much for him. At least he was able to see Avery home from the hospital and doing well. He had the opportunity to hold Avery and Mom even took a picture of them. I never thought about it until now, but that photo will be the only picture we'll ever have of Avery and Dad together.

I hate the turn of events life has thrown at me, but it's out of my control. Up until recently, there weren't many things—or perhaps anything—I would've changed in my life. I wonder how many people, if given the opportunity, would go back in time and change anything about their life? At first I think many would. When I think about it a little more, I don't feel that it's a good idea to mess with fate. Just the same, I still want my old life back.

Breaking the news to Jesse about Dad is more painful than I thought it could have been. I know she doesn't know what death means, or even that it exists. How do you tell a three-year-old that they'll never see their favorite person in the world anymore? She's been through so much turmoil in these past months, she doesn't deserve this.

Early evening has come and I know I can't procrastinate telling Jesse any longer. I'm actually a little perplexed because Jesse normally asks to see Grandpa constantly throughout the day. I take her outside to the swings. As we slowly swing back and forth, I turn to look at her and try to remain calm as I tell her Grandpa isn't going to be with us anymore, and we won't be able to see him again. God has taken him to heaven.

She gives me a very confused look and asks, "Why?"

I'm barely able to hold back the tears when I reply, "I'm not sure, honey. But I do know he didn't have a choice, and he would have never left you if he didn't have to."

She points up and says, "Grandpa heaven sky."

I say, "Yes, and he's watching you right now."

She stares up into the sky and starts waving while she repeats several times, "Grandpa, come back."

I can't keep it together any longer, and before I crumble into pieces in front of her I run into my bedroom and sob uncontrollably into my pillow. Cam sees me run into the bedroom and comes to check on me. No words are spoken, but he lets his presence be known from the comfort of his hand gently rubbing my back. I lay there and cry until no more tears are left.

Steven, Tammy, and Mom stay the next few nights at our house. At any given time throughout the day the house is filled with visitors. My fridge isn't big enough to house all the food everyone brings. At times the company is a nice distraction, sitting around telling funny stories about Dad. There are quite a few stories about Dad's younger rebel years. I love to hear the story about when he and Mom were dating, and one night they drove a motorbike right through the house where a party was being held, just for kicks. What I find most amusing about that story is the grin and twinkle in the eyes of Dad's friends who tell it to me.

Another story that causes much laughter was the time his doctor was coming to the house to check his blood pressure so he could see how it was in his home environment. It was always so tremendously high at the doctor's office, so he wanted to see if it was any lower at home. Dad got the bright idea to make sure that his blood pressure would give a good reading, so a few hours prior to the appointment he took four times too many relaxation pills, unbeknownst to Mom. Then he and Mom went to the barn to clean the horse stalls. Dad was so zonked out that Mom found him asleep with his head in the horses' feed bucket. She had a very hard time getting him back to the house. When she finally did the doctor had just arrived and it didn't take him long to realize what my Dad had been trying to do.

Dad had been incredibly close to Grandma and loved her as his own Mom. They absolutely adored each other. I find comfort knowing that Grandma and Dad are together again.

Dad had said many times that he didn't want a funeral, so we have a small service with just our closest family and friends. There is a short eulogy delivered by a family friend who is a minister. We all come back to my house afterwards and eat, and do some more reminiscing.

July 25

Mom is holding up well. She talks about Dad a lot, and always in the present tense, like he's still here. Steven is doing okay too, though still in a bit of shock. For days now he has continued to say, "I can't believe he's gone."

Tracee comes over for a visit today. I think she cries more than me while we sit on the grass talking about losing Dad. We are sitting there talking about Dad when suddenly I say, "Tracee, you're not going to believe it!"

"What?" she asks.

I reach over a few inches from where my hand was leaning on the grass. "Look at this."

In disbelief she asks, "That isn't a four-leaf clover, is it?"

Slowly I nod. "Yes it is! I can't believe it!"

Tears stream down both our faces, with hysterical laughter following.

"He's still here, Tracee. He's still with me," I say.

She grins. "I know."

As I mentioned earlier, for over a year I had been experiencing unsettling feelings about my Dad from time to time. This fear gave me a desire to take more videos of Jesse and Dad. I knew that if he passed away while she was young, at least she'd always have the videos to remember him by. Unfortunately, I didn't get the opportunity to make many. However, I know I have enough to help Jesse to remember her Grandpa, and how much he loved her. It has been a week since Dad died and I decide I want Jesse to see the videos. She has been asking about him more frequently every day.

Cam doesn't want me to show her the videos because he feels it's too soon, but she's missing her Grandpa terribly and needs to see him.

After I start to play the tapes I don't think it's possible for my heart to be any more broken than it already is. Her eyes light up and her mouth drops open. She's mesmerized while watching the videos over and over again. When we try to turn them off she starts to cry. She watches them for hours until she falls asleep on the floor in front of the TV.

It's been a week since Dad has passed and Mom feels she is as ready as she will ever be to go home. Until now Penni has been going back to Mom's house to get some of her clothes and toiletries, and to feed the cat. I understand how Mom feels because I can't see myself going back anytime soon. How will she ever be able to sleep in their bed ever again? I'm sure she'll be sleeping in the spare room for a long time, if not for the rest of her days at that house.

It makes me think back to when I was a teenager and my Grandma gave me her beautiful antique bedroom suite. It was hand-carved out of oak. I asked her why she wanted to give it to me then, and she said she knew that if she died while she was in bed sleeping, I'd never sleep in it. She was probably right. I slept in that bed for many years, and still have the bedroom suite today in my old bedroom at Mom's. It's the one Mom will probably be sleeping in.

I suggest to Mom she should move in with us, or we can buy a house with a suite. She said she appreciates the thought, but loves her home and wants to go back. I understand and somehow I know she's going to be okay. Although she had been with Dad since she was fourteen, I know that over time she will adjust. She may have been a former beauty queen but she is resilient and strong.

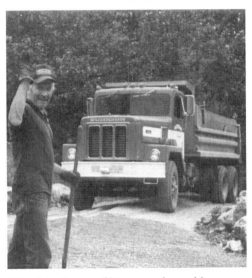

(Dad in front of his gravel truck)

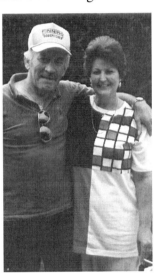

(Mom and Dad)

Chapter 12
A Visit With Dr. Human

July 26

We have been at home with Avery for a few weeks, but it's time to go back to Children's Hospital for a scheduled visit with Dr. Human to check out Avery's progress. I find it strange to be looking forward to seeing Dr. Human, but I kind of miss him. He's my larger-than-life hero, next to Avery. I'm definitely not looking forward to going back to the hospital, but I am a little curious to find out Dr. Human's thoughts on how Avery is doing. We feel he's doing great, but hearing it from a doctor will strengthen my peace of mind.

When we enter the parking lot of Children's Hospital a powerful rush of memories stir my emotions. So much has happened since the day we left this place that I have almost forgotten the familiar feeling of the fear which is now rapidly returning. My clenched fists begin to perspire and my heart races.

After we do the routine weigh-in, echo cardiogram, and ECG, we wait for Dr. Human in his office. Avery is undaunted by all the fuss, looking around the room full of smiles. When Dr. Human comes in, he's delighted to see Avery and how good he looks. Following a little chit chat, he brings out his stethoscope and checks him out.

Once he's finished, Dr. Human looks through Avery's chart then takes a second look at the earlier test results. With a pleased smile, he looks up at us and says everything appears to be great. He feels all systems are a 'go' for Avery's next heart surgery. Before I have a chance to digest his words, he explains that his receptionist, June, will be calling us in the next few days with a date and instructions. He anticipates that surgery will take place in the next couple of weeks.

The reality of it suddenly hits me: Avery will have to endure another surgery. I know it sounds crazy, but I had this hope (or rather fantasy) that we would go back to the hospital and Dr. Human would say that a miracle had taken place and Avery's heart had repaired itself. Perhaps it's this kind of wishful thinking that allows me to cope and keep some measure of sanity. However, no such luck. Yes, Avery is stronger and more stable since his last two operations, but the next surgeries are imminent.

When we shake hands and say our goodbyes, Dr. Human tells us what a wonderful job we've done taking care of Avery, and how babies with a loving family tend to thrive. It's the first time I realize how proud I am of Cam and I, and the tenacity we possess. So many times we could have cracked under the pressure, completely falling apart, and been no good to each other. Instead we make a terrific team.

As we dress Avery and gather our stuff, I feel the chill from the silence in the room. From the look on Cam's face, I know his thoughts echo mine: *Time to brace ourselves for Avery's next fight.*

Bonnie is working today and takes her break with us as we get a bite to eat before we leave. Thank goodness for Bonnie—or "Auntie

Bonnie" as she refers to herself when talking to Avery. She's going to make sure to be scheduled as Avery's nurse the day of his surgery. This is a big comfort for Cam and I. She knows Avery so well, and her close bond with him provides a huge relief to me.

The drive home is melancholic. Avery sleeps most of the way and Cam and I don't say too much. I'm trying to face the realization that Avery will be back in ICU in a couple of weeks, and accept the reality that we have a long road ahead.

Chapter 13
I Don't Like July Anymore

July 27

It's my thirty-second birthday, but I decide I don't like July any more. My Grandma died in July shortly before my birthday, and now my Dad. I don't really want to celebrate my birthday at all, but my mom thinks it's a good idea to try, so she prepares a big dinner for the family at her house.

It's my first birthday without my dad, but also the first time I'll go to their house since he died.

Pulling into their driveway is painful. Dad's big red gravel truck is sitting there, and I can see him in it, giving me a big smile and a thumbs up like he's done so many times before as I passed him on the road.

No sooner does the car stop when Jesse jumps out and begins running around the yard calling, "Grandpa! Grandpa!" She looks in the garage and anyplace else she has found him before. I wish I could be anywhere else in the world at this moment. She spots Dad's lawn mower, the one he had taken her for so many rides on. She jumps on it as she looks up into the sky (which she believes to be heaven and Dad's new home) and starts yelling, "Grandpa, ride! Come, peas!"

I fight back the tears and try again to explain that Grandpa can't come back anymore. I can tell she doesn't understand, but I don't know a way to make her understand.

Cam manages to talk Jesse into coming inside the house. Little do we know how much *more* painful this will be. She goes into every room of the house calling his name. Part of me wants to stop her, but I realize it may be best for her to check every room, allowing her to realize for herself that he isn't here.

Finding it difficult to breathe, I go outside for some fresh air and find Steven sitting on the steps—the same steps I sat on with Dad after Sam had died. Jesse's actions today are too much for Steven as well. He stares solemnly into the open field, deep in thought, and doesn't notice me until I sit down beside him and give him a big hug. We start talking about how bad the timing of all this is. After a few minutes of sitting there quietly watching the trees sway in the warm evening breeze, a strange feeling comes upon me. I put my hand on his shoulder and ask, "Are you thinking what I'm thinking?"

He clears his throat and with a quiet, hoarse voice he asks, "What are you thinking?"

Worried that I would sound like I've lost my mind, I hesitantly ask, "Do you ever wonder if Dad died so Avery could live?"

After a short pause, he lifts his head and with teary eyes he replies, "I do wonder that."

I don't how life actually works, but we know Dad would have given up his life for any one of his children. There is no doubt in my mind.

Under the circumstances, we make the best out of my birthday celebration. Mom cooks an amazing dinner, as she always has, with a homemade birthday cake and all.

After dinner, while everyone is eating dessert, I sneak into Mom and Dad's bedroom. As I sit on their bed and look around, I remember all the times I had become scared in the middle of the night and crawled into bed with them. I laugh when I think about how Dad always slept with his toes sticking out from under the sheets, and I would sometimes come home late at night and tickle his toes, almost sending him through the roof. I open his closet, and see his favorite white and red ski jacket. I picture the last time I saw him wearing it as I take in a deep breath of his scent.

I notice Dad's shiny yellow and black electric guitar nestled in the corner of his closet. He had played it for Steven and I so many times, singing his country songs. I vividly remember us sitting on the end of the bed as he would sing us his favorite country songs.

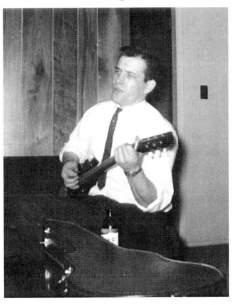

(Dad singing and playing guitar)

How lucky we are to have such memories.

Fifty-nine was too young to die, but I am grateful he had that much time. I just came from spending more than a month watching little babies die, seeing parents who would have begged, borrowed, or stole in order to have even one more day with their child. I know this all too well: I am one of them. I am glad I don't felt cheated. Instead I'm filled with gratitude to have been blessed with a wonderful relationship with my incredible dad.

Chapter 14

I Know My Grandma's Still With Me

August 3

There isn't much time to grieve the loss of Dad. We have to get ready for Avery's next surgery. It's scheduled for early morning on August 4, so today we pack all our clothes and head back to the hospital. It's probably a blessing in disguise. Having all this other stuff to deal with helps to take my mind off my sorrow.

Because we're going to be in ICU again, Cam's dad is bringing the motor home back to the parking lot at the hospital. I'm desperately hoping this time our ICU stay won't be for long. I wonder, *Am I delusional? Or am I starting to learn that optimism is the only glimmer of hope I have to keep me sane?* After all that has happened this past crazy couple of months I feel my life is out of control, like I'm watching a movie and yearning for a happy ending.

Mom comes this afternoon for a little visit before we go and to take Jesse home with her. Jesse's somber mood deepens while she watches me pack. She doesn't leave my side all day and keeps saying, "I come too." Again my explanation for leaving fails to make any sense to her.

My heart is broken beyond repair as I once again leave behind an inconsolable Jesse, and face the fear of the days ahead. It must be particularly difficult for Mom to say goodbye. We have seen her every single day since Dad died. She's putting on a brave face, but I wonder if she's merely holding on by threads. At least she'll have Jesse to keep her company.

Early evening we pull into the hospital's back parking lot where all the RVs stay. I notice that many have left and new ones have taken their place. It's a sad thought to realize that there will always be new ones filling the spot of the old ones. So much has happened since the last time we stayed in the motor home, but when we walk in, it certainly doesn't feel like six weeks have gone by.

It's a lovely summer evening and I want to savor every minute we have with Avery before surgery the next day. We sit outside on a blanket and watch the sunset. As my eyes follow the sun slowly disappearing behind the mountains, I realize that life stops for no one. I have been blessed to bring Avery home, and I'm more fortunate than many parents who would not ever have the opportunity to bring their baby home. Still, I want and need more: I want a lifetime with Avery.

I'm doing my best to stay positive, but tonight the fear is becoming overwhelming. I take Cam's hand in mine to draw some strength from his touch, but I know from the look on his face that his strength is waning as well.

As we pack up our stuff to head back to the motor home, I am in shock with what I discover. As I'm lifting the blanket off the ground to fold it up, I catch a glimpse of what I think is a four-leaf clover. It can't be! My eyes have fooled me before. But, sure enough, as I get closer I see that it is indeed. Even with the evening's warmth, goose bumps cover my body. I know it's a message from my Grandma! This is the fourth four-leaf clover I had found in two months! Unbelievable! Here we are, sitting on a tiny patch of grass beside the motor home in the hospital parking lot, and I find another four-leaf clover. My Grandma is telling me in the only way she can that she's here with us, watching over and protecting us.

Chapter 15
Here We Go Again

Surgery is bumped today because there are no available beds in ICU. Although it has delayed the inevitable, I'm happy that it gives us an extra day to spend with Avery. It's only one more guaranteed day, but to me it's worth its weight in gold.

Dr. LeBlanc doesn't appear happy to tell us the news about postponing Avery's surgery. He knows we just want to get it over with.

During our last visit to see him, Dr. LeBlanc explained what this surgery would entail, but it sounded so complicated, so this morning I ask him to explain it again. This is what he says, "I will be performing a pulmonary artery band (literally a band closing off the blood supply to the pulmonary artery), and a BT shunt (redirecting the blood flow). This surgery is a necessary step before the open heart surgery because it will allow Avery's body to slowly adjust to the big switch, when the great arteries are cut off and switched. Without this surgery, Avery's system would be overwhelmed with the extreme change in blood flow, causing a great potential to die of a heart attack."

Oh boy, I am sorry I asked.

Check-in is 6:30 in the morning. We stand at the window in front of surgical daycare, and a stone-faced nurse tells us to go to room three, gown Avery, and wait. She is so cold and methodical. Maybe she's a good nurse, but it wouldn't have hurt to throw in a little compassion. She probably never knew the feeling of having to hand over her own baby to have its heart operated on. If she had, she'd have known the desperate fear a parent feels, and would've been more comforting.

It's a long wait in a tiny cubicle because surgery isn't scheduled until 8:30 a.m. For the most part, Avery is calm and peaceful, giving us smiles, especially when I sing to him. He starts to get cranky towards the end of the wait, and I can't blame him. He's hungry, and hasn't been allowed to nurse since midnight. He has become used to nursing every couple hours, developing a voracious appetite.

Bonnie briefly stops in to say "Hi" and to confirm that she'll be Avery's nurse after surgery. I'm so grateful for Bonnie and her fondness for Avery. Something about him touches her soul. This lets me know he'll be in the best care with her.

As surgery draws near my anxiety intensifies. Soon some nurse I have never seen before will come and take Avery from my arms.

I pass the time by watching the other parents sitting with their babies. Some are waiting for surgery for a broken limb, and others for major dental surgery requiring sedation. No matter what the reason, I can see fear in their eyes. I am dreadfully afraid too; my son is about to have heart surgery right after a heart attack killed my beloved father. If I didn't know that this was happening to me,

I'd never believe it. I feel life has swallowed me up in some kind of vortex.

It's about 8:00 a.m. when a young, soft-spoken nurse walks up to us and checks Avery's tags, confirming we're the Gemmells then tells us Dr. LeBlanc is ready for Avery. She says surgery will take about three hours, and we'll be paged when it's over. She makes it sound so simple, like I was handing over a pair of pants to get hemmed, and she'd call me when they were ready.

Passing Avery to her is even more painful than I had imagined. He looks at me with a big smile so trustingly. I feel a tightening in the pit of my stomach. For a second I think of turning and running away with him in my arms. At least then I would be guaranteed a little more time with him. By giving him to the nurse, there are no guarantees of sharing any more time.

But I know what I have to do. I delicately place Avery in her arms, and pray it won't be the last time I see him alive. I try to push any negative thoughts away, but I can't ignore the possibility. The nurse slowly walks away down the hall corridor with Avery in her arms. I watch until they pass through the big swinging doors marked with large print that reads, *Patients Only*. I hug Cam tightly for many minutes, and cry.

In our silence, Cam and I are doing our best to hold it together when Dr. LeBlanc, dressed in his blue scrubs and a colorful hat, comes into the parents' waiting area. I'm glad to see him, and had hoped for an opportunity to talk to him before he operated on Avery. He says, "I just saw Avery and he looks great. You guys have done a terrific job with him at home. It's nice to see such a healthy weight gain on him. I will take good care of him this morning, and will be seeing you in a few hours."

I have so many questions for him, but wouldn't you know it, my mind goes totally blank. I just stand there nodding my head, and before I can articulate any of my thoughts, he's gone.

Dr. LeBlanc's compliment on Avery's terrific progress feels good, especially since he's a man of few words. Little does he know how challenging things have been for us at home. The compliment helps me to realize that I have done my little part to help save my baby's life. For so much of this ordeal I've felt completely helpless.

Once again, the wait is on. It is déjà vu. Just like before, we sit in almost complete silence, trying to endure the pain in our hearts. I keep looking at the pager in my hand to see if I have missed a call. I try to read magazines to pass the time, but the words don't register. I try counting the heartbeats pounding loudly in my chest, but that doesn't work either. It only makes me think of Avery's little heart, and him fighting for his life. Cam and I watch the clock, somehow managing to say a few words of encouragement to each other every now and again.

It occurs to me that this time is a little different than the last surgery, because now not only does Avery have Grandma working in his corner, he has my Dad too. I know if he has any opportunity to help from heaven he'll be doing whatever he can. He'll be pulling a "Sam," telling God to make a bionic kid out of Avery if He has to!

My thoughts are scattered and make no sense. And why is time passing so darn slowly? It feels like there are a thousand minutes to every hour. A few hours have passed and still we hear nothing. One after the other, worried thoughts spin through my head like a whirlwind while fragments of speculations pierce through me like shattered glass.

Just like the last surgery, I feel my composure slipping. I'm becoming desperate as I tell Cam, "They should be finished by now! I'm going to ICU to find…." Just then the door opens and Dr. LeBlanc walks in. I jump up but my flimsy legs buckle. I try again and this time I succeed. As he approaches I look to find some emotion on his face to tell me the answer. I think I see a faint look of optimism hiding behind his stern unshaven face, but I don't want to get my hopes up, so I impatiently wait for him to speak.

Dr. LeBlanc states confidently, "Surgery went well."

My mouth drops open and I turn to look at Cam. I literally see color fill his pale face along with a look of welcome relief begin to emerge.

Dr. LeBlanc tells us everything went as planned with no surprises. Avery is being stabilized in ICU, and we'll be able to see him in a few minutes.

Wow! He's just finished operating on my son's heart, and makes it sound like it's as routine as waiter serving a bowl of soup without spilling it. Does he have any idea of the enormous admiration and gratitude parents like us feel after an ordeal of this magnitude? I don't even know how to begin to convey my feelings to him. For the time being all I can think of is to give him a big hug and to thank him profusely. Thank goodness he's a big man or the strength of my hug might have squished the 'stuffing' out of him. Cam gives a hearty pat-on-the-back man hug, with many thanks as well.

Walking around the corner to ICU is all too familiar. This time, however, I thought it would have been easier because I knew what to expect. It wasn't all that long ago we had been down this road. But I'm wrong. I don't think it ever gets easier when your baby is this sick.

Approaching ICU, I can hear the blinging and dinging of the monitors. There is a crowd of doctors and nurses surrounding Avery's bed. Dr. Human walks up to us and reiterates Dr. LeBlanc's words regarding the success of the surgery. He mentions a little concern about Avery's high heart beat and fluctuating blood oxygen saturations, but thinks this will stabilize over the next few hours.

It's difficult to see Avery hooked up to life support and all the other wires and machines again. Just a few hours ago he had been smiling at me and making cute noises. Now he's lying unconscious with a machine doing the breathing for him, keeping him alive. All the desperate and helpless feelings return with a vengeance, making it hard to breathe. I need to sit down. Tears fill my eyes. Cam sits quietly on the stool fighting back his tears, never taking his eyes off Avery and the monitors reading his vital signs.

Thank goodness Bonnie is Avery's nurse today! As soon as she can spare a moment from stabilizing Avery, she comes to give us a big hug, assuring us that things are going as expected, and telling us she'll ensure they stay that way.

The rest of the day is pretty bumpy. Avery's heart rate still hasn't stabilized yet, and his low oxygen saturations tell us he's struggling. The 7:00 p.m. shift change is approaching, and I don't want Bonnie to go, but am relieved when I see Diane arrive and she tells us that she is Avery's nurse for the night shift. As much as I would have preferred Bonnie to stay, I know she's exhausted and needs a good night's sleep. Diane is shocked to see how much Avery has grown. She has taken care of him before, but hasn't seen him since he was three weeks old.

Again all night and early into the morning, we sit in a hypnotic state watching Avery sleep, trying not to let the unstable, fluctuating monitors displaying his vital signs magnify our worry. Diane manages to convince Cam and I to go and get a few hours sleep. As she so eloquently says in her New Zealand accent, "You guys look *awful*! Go get some sleep. I'll call you if anything changes."

I wake early, my heart racing with anticipation. Cam barely gets his clothes on as I pull him out the door. Running to ICU feels like a dream where I can't go fast because cement shoes are weighing down my feet. I keep thinking things must be okay because we haven't received any phone calls to tell us otherwise. As I turn the familiar corner to ICU, I spot Bonnie at Avery's bedside displaying a look of concern. *Oh no*, I thought. *Here we go again!*

She explains that Avery's heart rate is still high, and he hasn't peed since before surgery. He is in renal failure, and the doctors are worried his kidneys are shutting down.

Oh God, let this be a bad dream, I think. *We've been through enough. Avery has been through way too much.*

All day nothing changes, and in the evening Dr. Adderley decides to hook Avery up to the dialysis machine in order to help him pee. It is a crucial time. Avery needs to pee by the next day or his kidneys likely won't recover. What does this mean? A kidney transplant? Or even worse? I can't handle what the answer may be, so I don't ask the question. It's killing me to sit here unable to do anything to help this newest setback. Again, Cam and I helplessly watch as Avery fights for his life.

Convinced I can't helplessly sit here anymore, an idea pops into my head, and I run up to the library to find a book on reflexology. I find a chart where all the organs of the body are displayed on the foot. Many naturopathic doctors—and some conventional doctors—believe that the nerve endings of all body organs are in the feet, and that massaging the problem area can stimulate and assist in healing. I wasn't sure of this, but I had to try. I look at the foot chart, find where the kidneys are located, and run back to ICU to try my naturopathic approach.

I start gently massaging the bottom of his feet, first the left, then the right. After about a half hour, I notice the doctors are starting to make their rounds. When they arrive at Avery's bed, their faces take on puzzled looks. Dr. Adderley asks me what I'm doing, so I explain my reflexology attempt. He looks at me like I'm some kind of voodoo doctor. I don't care. I'm a desperate mom, grasping at straws to try to save my newborn baby.

It's late into the evening and no pee yet. I can't bear sitting here waiting anymore. Close to state of delirium, we listen to Diane's advice to try and get a couple hours sleep. Yeah, like *that's* possible. All I manage to do is toss and turn while all kinds of different scenarios play out in my mind.

August 7

About 6:00 a.m., my cell phone rings. I literally throw it at Cam like a fastball pitch. The lump forming in my throat is so big I'm not capable of answering. Cam answers and almost immediately looks relieved. I hear him say, "Thanks Bonnie. This is such great news! We're on our way down. See you in a few minutes."

Cam gets off the phone and shouts, "Avery just took a pee! Bonnie is so excited I could barely understand what she was saying. She came to work early because she was so worried about Avery and couldn't sleep anyway."

"Thank God! Thank God!" is all I can manage to say as I scramble to get my shoes on.

Within seconds we're racing through the parking lot down to ICU. I'm wearing my PJs and slippers, and my messy hair is flying all over the place.

Yes, Avery has managed to jump over another hurdle. No doubt I'm excited, but scared at the same time. How many more hurdles will he have to jump? How much more can his little body take? Is the worst over now? Only time will unfold any answers, but for now, I must remain focused on today and this little victory.

I do wonder, and always will, if my reflexology treatment had anything to do with it. I'm definitely leaning towards a "yes."

August 9

Fortunately, the past few days have been fairly uneventful. Avery is stabilizing nicely and we are having lots of visits from friends and family. I also have had some time to catch up with most of our hospital neighbors.

Tina is not doing well at all. She's in severe kidney and renal failure. It has been days since she had a bowel movement or passed any urine. Dialysis doesn't seem to be working, and the outlook is bleak. Lisa and Ben look more haggard than ever. They sit at Tina's bedside not speaking much to anyone except the doctors and nurses.

Noah hasn't been doing much better either. After many attempts he still hasn't been able to come off of life support, and his condition is much too delicate to perform the heart surgery he needs. His mom displays more of a desperate defeated look with every passing day. We try to keep her company as much as possible, and provide some encouragement.

The tenacity and compassion of humans continues to amaze me. We are all are going through our own crises, yet we somehow still find the strength to provide support to others in similar or worse situations.

Little Taylor appears to be doing the same as he was when we left for our brief stay at home. His parents are frustrated because he isn't successfully coming off of life support. He sits up in bed most of the day, with his parents next to him, coloring and watching the action going on around him. I can't imagine what he must be feeling or thinking. Even though he's now back at the hospital, I keep thinking how lucky his parents were to have had him at home, living a normal happy life for the past three years. I know it doesn't seem like a whole lot of time to most people, but compared to the chance that you may *never* get to take your baby home, it seems to be plenty.

Today I find out that while we were at home with Avery, Anthony's parents finally decided to listen to the doctors, remove his life support, and let him go. After the doctors removed the breathing tubes from Anthony, the parents and extended family sat around his bed with outbursts of cries while waiting for the monitor to flat line, but it never did. The family thought it was a miracle, but the doctors and nurses knew otherwise. They had seen this many times before. Because Anthony had been on life support for so long, his body semi-healed, but his brain hadn't. He was considered alive but 'brain dead.' He was moved to another ward in the hospital. Hopefully in the next few days I'll be able to find his parents and see how they're doing.

Chapter 16
All Systems Go

It's been a few days since Avery's renal failure episode, and the doctors are starting to talk about extubating him. It's weird: a couple months ago I had never heard of the word "extubate," but now it's a staple in our vocabulary.

Avery continues to improve and has a good chance for a successful extubation, but Dr. LeBlanc wants to wait a couple more days because of the failed attempts from the other surgeries. It's quite apparent that whatever Dr. LeBlanc says to do is what the ICU doctors do, even if they don't agree.

I'm okay with waiting because providing Avery with more time to gain strength makes sense to me. Some nurses feel doctors move things along a little too quickly in order to free the beds for incoming patients who have been on long wait lists for surgery. It doesn't seem fair any way I look at it, but it is what it is. The extra time waiting also gives me an opportunity to go to Chilliwack for a visit with Jesse. I know she must be crushed. Her Grandpa is gone, and her Mom, Dad, and brother have left her too. It's not possible to imagine what she must be feeling.

When I pull into Mom and Dad's driveway I can see Jesse's pretty little face peer out the window then quickly disappear. Next thing I know she's running out the door with arms outstretched, ready for the biggest hug. Mom follows, and we all share a group hug. Mom says Jesse is doing well, considering that the other day she said, "Grandpa, Mommy, Daddy, Avery, all gone." Mom told her, "Yes, Grandpa is gone, but Mommy, Daddy, and Avery will be coming back."

It's too difficult to bring Jesse home because I know she won't want to leave, and it will only prolong the dreadful goodbye. So we stay at Mom's, enjoying a few precious hours together. I do my best to erase all other things on my mind in order to focus only on my time with Jesse, but my heart aches. It aches because I know I'll have to leave Jesse again, and she needs me so much right now. It aches because I feel guilty being away from my son, who is fighting for his life. It aches because I don't know how much more I can take. And it aches because I miss Dad terribly.

When early evening comes, my urge to return to the hospital escalates. Cam had called earlier and said to take my time, that Avery is doing fine, but I need to be by his side.

It progressively gets more difficult to say goodbye to Jesse, and this time I take the coward's way out by waiting until she's asleep then sneaking off. I carefully pry her sleeping body from my arms and place her in Grandma's bed, gently gliding her hair off her face and saying goodbye with a soft kiss on her forehead. She looks so perfect that it is difficult to take my eyes off her. I wish I could sit here all night watching her peaceful sleep.

Trying to be strong for Mom's sake, I fight back the tears as we say our goodbyes. But once I get in my car the floodgates unleash, blurring my vision. I have to pull over down the road and let the tears fall until they run dry.

When I regain enough composure, I continue the drive back and begin daydreaming about the day I'll be sitting in my backyard with Avery in my arms and watching Jesse on the swings.

We make a choice about what we imagine or what we think, so I choose to think good thoughts. It will certainly help me more than thinking negative ones. Thinking positively helps the spirit, but sometimes when devastation is everywhere it's impossible to stay positive.

I know that Cam said Avery is doing great, but until I see him sleeping peacefully in his bed I won't be able to feel any sense of calm. It's late in the evening when I arrive back at ICU, and Cam has already left to get a good night's sleep for a change. Linda says he had been falling asleep in the chair. I stay and chat with Linda while I hold Avery for a couple of hours. It's been a mentally exhausting day, yet a good one.

August 11

The morning rounds confirm all systems are a go for extubation this morning. Cam and I go to get a cup of coffee during the procedure, and by the time we return, Avery is breathing on his own. What a beautiful sight. Avery's face once again is clear of any tubes and wires. He's a little fussy, but we know that's to be expected. Apparently, when the tubes come out, the throat is very scratchy and sore. As the day progresses, Avery seems to be breathing with ease, much more easily than his last extubation. He hasn't been demonstrating any stress at all, and looks comfortable. Another great day and one day closer to bringing him home. It feels good to feel optimism and hope again. I know the tug of war isn't over, but at least we're on the winning side for now.

August 12

This morning Dr. Human comes to check on Avery, and is very pleased. He informs us that the plan is for Avery to go to the observation ward tomorrow for a few days, then home for a few weeks, and then the final open heart surgery. It's nice to see a smile on Dr. Human's face while he explains the plan. With all the unexpected curve balls Avery has thrown our way, I'm sure Dr. Human is quite thrilled we have arrived at this juncture. He also states that this recent surgery has been more challenging on Avery's body than the Switch will be. I ask why and he replies, "When we do the Switch, Avery's heart will finally be fixed and he'll most likely thrive."

August 13

Avery is continuing to impress the doctors with his progress. He's full of smiles, and needless to say, so are we. At about 11:15 a.m., we say our goodbyes to the ICU staff, and off we go to the third floor. Once we settle into the room, I decide to go pump some milk. Avery's throat has been too sore to breastfeed so I need to keep pumping to provide my milk through the NG feeding tube.

I'm on my way back with two full bottles of milk, smiling to myself and feeling so good about things, when all of a sudden I hear what sounds like a herd of elephants running, closing in behind me. I turn my head to see a team of doctors dashing towards me at ninety miles an hour. A Code Blue has been called!

A chill races through my veins as I watch them run past me and turn the corner. I think, *Please! Don't turn right!* But they do. I pick up my pace and as I turn the corner I say to myself, *Don't turn left!* But they do. *Oh no! They can't be going to Avery's room! He's doing so well! What could have possibly happened in such a short time?* But when I turn left, I see the team of doctors has reached their destination. It's Avery's bed. The Code Blue has been called for him. He's in respiratory arrest.

Chapter 17
Code Blue

All my self control vanishes in an instant. I collapse to the ground, my milk crashing to the floor, and I begin hyperventilating. Bonnie and another nurse run to me. I am hysterical, screaming, and violently shaking my head from side to side. No one can calm me. I have "hit the wall" and am ready for a straitjacket. Bonnie can't think of anything else to do but slap me in the face. This stops the hyperventilating, but now all I can do is sit on the floor, rocking, repeatedly asking, "Is he dead? Is he dead?"

I hear someone say, "No, the doctors are working on him right now."

I notice Cam coming out of the room looking as white as a ghost, unable to speak. We slump in silence on the floor in the hallway while the team of doctors works on our baby. We don't know if we'll ever see Avery alive again.

Mrs. Johnston's message from God echoes in my head. I again remind myself of the four-leaf clovers I had found, and their significance. It doesn't matter. No amount of positive thinking can help me now—only Avery's survival can. I have just lost my Dad. God can't possibly take Avery from me too.

Through tears and broken sentences, Cam begins telling Bonnie and me what happened leading up to Avery's arrest. He says Avery had started to get really fussy, escalating to an uncontrollable scream. Cam noticed his heart rate was dropping rapidly on the monitor, so he screamed for the nurse, "Something is wrong! Call Dr. Human!" Cam pauses. "I was so mad. The nurse didn't seem to sense the urgency. She took her time to respond. When she finally made her way over and saw the severity of the situation, she immediately called a Code Blue." Cam's voice chokes even more but he manages to finally get the words out, "But by the time the doctors got there, Avery was . limp in my arms."

He doesn't say it, but I know Cam fears the worst.

Finally, Dr. LeBlanc comes into the hallway to see us. He explains that Avery is intubated and back on life support. He needs to go back to ICU and to do some tests and try to determine the reason for his crash. He adds, "Avery is in critical condition. You need to brace yourselves for a stormy patch ahead."

Part of me is dead, but the tattered part remaining is grateful he's still alive. A coping mechanism hibernating in the depths of my body emerges. Avery is still with us. There's still hope. *Grandma and Dad must be providing me with the strength to carry on, because I don't think I can do it on my own.*

I am in the midst of trying to endure the magnificent pain life can sometimes deliver. Whenever I think about atrocities such as the Holocaust, I'm in awe of people's will to survive such devastating circumstances. I've never been able to fathom their will to continue. Even though our situation is completely different, I have a slightly better understanding now.

My little precious baby, how much more can your body take? I want you to know how proud we are of you. I want you to know what an incredible fighter you are. I need you to live so I can tell you how much you're loved.

The past couple days have been unbearable. I'm numb from head to toe, and how I'm functioning is beyond me. I feel like I'm in a horrible movie or nightmare that just keeps replaying. Avery's condition is so weak that he has to be administered a paralyzing drug every couple of hours in order to keep him from another arrest. Our instructions are to stare at him closely and wait for him to start moving. When he starts to twitch the nurse gives him another needle to keep him paralyzed. He can't be moved, and holding him is out of the question. Changing his diaper is as dicey as defusing a bomb. He's even developed a bed sore at the back of his head because he can't be shifted in the slightest.

I tell everyone that I don't want visitors. I can barely muster the strength to talk to the nurses and doctors, let alone anyone else. I talk to Mom at least twice today, but I can't pretend like I'm doing okay. Cam isn't doing much better. His face looks sad and defeated. I'm sure a part of him died when Avery went limp in his arms. It will be impossible to forget that experience. The only thing that will provide any solace is for Avery to show some improvement.

This is horrible timing for Dr. Human to be taking a week off, although he surely needs and deserves a break. I've heard that he hasn't gone out of town, so I find a phone book and look up his number. I keep it on a piece of paper in my pocket, and continually contemplate phoning him.

Dr. LeBlanc and the ICU doctors are uncertain about what's going on with Avery. His lungs are wet, so they're hoping that the Lacix (furosemide) they've administered will dry them out. Dr. Adderley has been adjusting his meds in attempts to help stabilize him. All we can do is wait and see if anything the doctors have done will work.

This morning I phone Mrs. Johnston to pray. I tell her what has been happening and she says Avery needs to be "anointed with oil." I'm scared when she tells me this because I think anointing is something a priest does just before a person dies. However, it's not that at all. The purpose of anointing Avery is to give him strength, joy, and peace. It's also part of a Biblical procedure when praying for someone's healing. So we arrange for a chaplain to come from a church in Vancouver to perform the anointing.

The next day, a very tall, thin man in his late fifties comes. He's gentle and kind, with a soft-spoken voice. We stand around Avery's bed while the chaplain prays and rubs some kind of oil on Avery's forehead. It's a surreal moment, and extremely emotional. Everything is so overwhelming. The world as I know it no longer exists. I don't know anything anymore.

A couple days pass and no change. It's the morning of Dr. Human's return from holidays, at around 6:30 a.m. I begin to wait for his arrival at his office door. Sitting on the floor with my back resting against the wall, I must have fallen into a light slumber because the next thing I know I'm being awakened by Dr. Human greeting me a "Good morning." His face fills with compassion as I jump up and begin to ramble, trying to explain the latest turn of events. Emotion and tears get the best of me, and I'm too distraught to enunciate words. Dr. Human gives me a big hug and tells me that he's abreast of Avery's situation. He tells me, "I have called every day to check on Avery's condition, and to discuss treatment with Dr. LeBlanc. I believe we are taking the correct course of action, but we will have to wait and see." His words don't bring much relief, but his return from holidays is a much-needed reassurance.

It has been a few days and Avery is starting to show slight signs of improvement. Mrs. Johnston appears to know what he needed. The chaplain's anointing must have worked. Avery's vital signs are becoming more stable, and he's able to come off the paralyzing drug. His lungs have dried out and the adjustments to his medicine appear to be working well. It has been four days since Avery's arrest, and he's finally able to open his eyes again. This is another miracle.

Bonnie and Avery's other nurses are in complete awe of him. They can't believe his resiliency and strength to keep fighting. These improvements bring tremendous relief but I'm petrified to think what lies ahead. There's still another major open heart surgery around the corner. I try to focus on only one day at a time, yet the fear sometimes finds its way in. I want to be optimistic, but our experiences thus far make it difficult.

We are into the middle of August, and the heat is making it difficult to sleep. That, coupled with our worries, makes for little or no sleep. Last night we did manage to get a bit of sleep, but I had the worst nightmare of my life. I dreamed we had taken Avery home, all fixed and totally healthy. We were at home celebrating and having a great time when Avery suddenly started convulsing and stopped breathing. I yelled, "Call 911! Call 911!" at the top of my lungs. It was such a vivid dream.

I yelled so loud that it woke us up immediately. I asked Cam, "Did I just yell out, 'Call 911'?"

He answered, "Oh yes, and it was very loud." We started laughing hysterically because all the windows were open, and there must have been at least ten other RVs all around us. Because it was so hot, I was sure they had their windows open too. We lay there for a long time quietly giggling while we wondered if we'd be hearing the sound of sirens coming our way. It was a terrible dream, but it sure felt good to laugh. I can't wait for the day when laughter is a daily part of my life again, if indeed it's possible.

Chapter 18
Hope Returns

August 19

Avery continues to show improvement, and so do my spirits. My outlook is starting to heal from this latest blow, and I'm finally able to have conversations with people other than Cam again. I feel no hesitation to pour out my feelings to the other parents here. We're all in the same vulnerable position and intimately know each other's pain. I especially like Taylor's dad, Gord, and his optimism. I feel so bad for him and Cynthia. I can see their frustration really starting to grow, and I can't blame them. Taylor has had many failed attempts coming off life support. Now Gord says there is talk about Taylor needing a heart transplant. They retain hope but are growing more worried with every passing day. It's scary for me when I think Avery has the same defect as Taylor.

I can also understand Ben and Lisa's frustration. Bonnie tells me that Tina has been moved to the isolation room. The doctors have given her only a couple of days to live. She's still in severe renal and kidney failure, and the doctors have run out of options. I just don't get it. If God is going to take Tina, why doesn't He do it right away? Why does she have to suffer so much, only to die?

I run into Lisa in the hallway and she just breaks down in front of me. I know how she feels, but there's nothing I or anyone can say that would help. I let her know about the reflexology I had done on Avery's feet to help stimulate his kidneys to pee. She says anything is worth a try at this point. We give each other a big hug and she tells me she'll keep me posted on Tina's condition.

The other day Bonnie told me she has a feeling that the doctors are wrong—Tina isn't going to die. She said she has no evidence to support her theory; it's just a feeling. I hope she's right.

Not long after Tina moves to the isolation room, a newborn baby with a heart defect moves into her space. All through the night the baby keeps having heart attacks, needing to be revived. The curtains close as the parents prepare for the worst. By morning when we return to ICU, the spot is empty. At the doctors' request, the parents signed a consent to a DNR (Do not resuscitate) because there was no quality of life left. The defect was too complex to be fixed. So that's what they did. How devastating! No parent should ever have to consent to let their child die ... and yet it happens all the time. I'm in a nightmare. Such travesties never existed before. Well, actually that isn't true ... they existed but never to me, until now.

I'm so lost and desperate, and sometimes I can't stop the dark scenarios that enter my mind. It's becoming increasingly difficult to not let these unending tragedies cripple my thinking. However, Avery is doing better, and I must just try to focus on that. Dr. LeBlanc is talking about trying to extubate Avery tomorrow. Over a week has passed since his arrest and he's been stable now for four days.

What will Avery have in store for us this time?

Dr. Human feels Avery is more than ready to come off of life support, but I'm sure he thought that *last* time too. My nerves are frazzled and my hands shake as Cam and I wait outside of ICU while Avery is being extubated. When it's time to see him I can hear him crying as we approach his bed. He's cranky because his poor little throat is so sore from all the tubes going in and out. I want to pick him up and console him but I'm not allowed to. So I gently stroke the top of his head while I watch the clock, hoping with all my might that Avery can succeed in breathing on his own this time.

Time passes at a painfully slow pace, but so far so good. Avery's stats remain strong throughout the day, with no sign of wavering. His heartbeat remains at a good resting rate. I'm cautiously optimistic that Avery is going to succeed in staying off life support this time. He looks so much better now than he did before his respiratory arrest.

If everything goes the way we hope, the plan is to go home for three to four weeks. Dr. Human feels this will give Avery extra time to adapt to the redirection of blood flow from his new band and shunt. Even though it will be a temporary visit home, a long-lost feeling of excitement returns.

My biggest worry is going back to the dreaded observation ward. The wounds from last time are too fresh. When I share my feeling with Dr. LeBlanc he says, "I can understand why. I'm not even his parent and it brings back bad memories for me."

Later in the day I'm surprised to learn from Bonnie that Dr. LeBlanc and Dr. Wensley (head of ICU) had words at the bedside. Dr. LeBlanc said he wanted Avery to be discharged from ICU and bypass the observation ward. Dr. Wensley said, "Fine, Jacques. Then we'll just cancel your surgeries for the next week because of lack of available beds." Bonnie then said Dr. LeBlanc replied, "He won't be here that long." Then he stormed off. Bonnie can't believe how Avery has affected everyone at the hospital, especially Jacques. "In my twelve years of being here, no one has ever gone home straight from ICU," she says with a raised eyebrow. I think it's because they have so much admiration for this little guy who keeps fighting and defying all odds."

Today is also a blessing for Lisa and Ben. Tina passed water in the morning, and then had a bowel movement in the afternoon. It's nothing short of a miracle. Bonnie was right: educated guess or sixth sense, I'm not sure which. Tina is still in critical condition, but this is wonderful news. Lisa is going around ICU like she's walking on clouds, telling everyone the good news. It's so nice to see a smile on her face. What a difference a smile can make on a person. Or should I say, what a difference a little good news can bring.

Chapter 19
Bittersweet

<u>August 21</u>

I can't believe the phone call I receive from Mom today! Jesse has been exposed to chicken pox from Tracee's son, Brett. Jesse had a sleepover there, and Brett woke up with full-blown chicken pox. This means that Jesse can be nowhere near Avery for a month. If Avery is exposed to chicken pox he won't be able to have his surgery. We're finally able to come home for a brief visit and to try to restore some normalcy to our lives, not to mention how tremendously excited I am to spend much-needed time with Jesse … and now she can't be with us.

I miss Jesse terribly, and this news is a big blow. Now I'll have to go to my Mom's house to visit Jesse, and then will have to leave her all over again. She's going to be devastated every time I leave without her. I'm worried all this upheaval in her life may cause some kind of emotional damage. How could it not?

It has been four days since Avery's extubation, and he's doing amazingly well. So after rounds this morning Avery is discharged from ICU. It's a day of mixed feelings. It's wonderful to be bringing Avery home, but so disappointing that Jesse can't be there waiting to greet us with that beautiful smile of hers.

On our way home, Cam drops Avery and me off and continues on to Mom's house for a visit with Jesse. Other than the furniture, my house looks vacant and abandoned with no sign of life. I quickly open all the windows and doors to get rid of the stuffiness and to let in some fresh air. Being in our backyard is so private that I decide to take Avery out into the warm, fresh air to feed him.

While I'm sitting outside nursing Avery, I stare out into the cow pasture, and am reminded of the day the farmer took the momma's newborn calf away from her, remembering how she went totally ballistic, attacking the farmer as he wheeled her little baby away. I hated the farmer at the time, and wished the cow would have knocked him down, but I knew it wasn't right. He was doing his job. That's how life works. I wonder if that cow ever recovered from her pain, and how many other calves were taken away from her.

I've been home about thirty minutes and I can't think of much else but seeing Jesse. As much as I can't wait to see her, I'm apprehensive because leaving Mom's without her might be more painful for her than not seeing her at all. I have to take that chance though. She needs me.

I just finish feeding Avery for the second time in less than a couple hours when Cam returns. He tells me how much Jesse begged to come with him and how the torture of leaving her behind made him cry all the way home. Cam decides to have a little nap with Avery, and I make my way to Mom's house. On my way there I think about what I'm going to tell Jesse. I decide that it's best not to tell her we're temporarily at home. It will be so much easier if she thinks we're still at the hospital. I hate to hide the truth from her, but I know she won't understand the whole chicken pox scare, and why she isn't able to come home with us.

As I drive into the driveway, I can see Jesse in the garden, picking peas. She doesn't see me, so I sit and watch her for a few minutes. She picks a pea pod, fusses to open it, spills most onto the ground, and yet manages to get a few in her mouth—then she starts all over. What an *ahhh* moment for me. It's simple, but almost magical. She's here, she's healthy, and she's my precious daughter.

As I watch I have to chuckle when I notice Grandma chide her for putting peas in her mouth that have fallen to the ground. Jesse doesn't like what Grandma has to say, and as she turns to walk away, she notices me in the driveway. With peas flying in the air, she runs to me as fast as her little legs can go.

It's a wonderful visit while we rummage through the garden for fresh carrots and peas. There are moments where I feel we've never been apart. Jesse seems very content as she stuffs peas into my mouth. Many are overripe, but how can I refuse her generosity?

Mom starts to mow the lawn. This is my first time seeing her on the big John Deere ride-on. It seems weird. Dad is supposed to be doing that. I'm so proud of Mom and how she's tackling widowhood. I wouldn't even have been able to start the lawn mower, and yet there she is carefully going back and forth, then crisscross, to create the perfect checkered pattern on the grass like Dad always did.

I smile while this reminds me of what a perfectionist Dad was. He wouldn't let anyone mow the lawn except for him because we didn't do it "just right." I was quite happy about that, but Steven, as a kid, thought the big lawn mower was a blast to ride on. I sure miss Dad. It's difficult coming here sometimes. There are so many wonderful memories, but I'm not ready to relish them yet.

It's a fulfilling visit with Jesse and Mom, and I'd like to stay longer, but after a few hours the two wet spots on my T-shirt tell me it's time to go home soon. Avery will be getting hungry.

It's so hard saying goodbye to Jesse, I don't know how I'll be able to do it. What is she thinking? When I leave she must be wondering how long before she'll see me again, if ever. Just when she probably starts to forget about me she gets her heart broken again when I return, only to leave her all over again. If only she were a little older she would have a better understanding. Then perhaps it would be less devastating for both of us. I want to scream. I want to grab her, put her in the car, and drive her home.

It has been such a great visit and I don't want to ruin it by another heart-wrenching departure, so once again, I take the coward's way out and sneak out after Jesse falls asleep for an afternoon nap. She looks so peaceful sleeping on the couch holding on to her little Sesame Street Ernie and Bert sock. That never leaves her hands. She carries it with her wherever she goes, probably because it's the only consistent thing her life possesses right now.

The tears are still rolling down my cheeks as I arrive home, but walking into the house and seeing Avery snuggling in Cam's arms instantly eases my anxiety. Despite missing Jesse, the three of us have a great evening. The best part is cuddling with Avery on the couch while Cam and I watch the movie *Titanic* for the first time. I'll forever be grateful for that movie. For the first time in months

I'm carried away from my turbulent life and lost in one of the greatest love stories of all time. It's a wonderful diversion, and I wish the movie wouldn't end. I want the distraction to continue so reality can be postponed a little longer.

After the movie ends, we get into bed with Avery between us. How lovely to be in our own bed again. As I lay here, I realize, due to pure exhaustion, that I haven't been faithful with my evening prayers for quite some time. I feel so many different emotions tonight that my prayer is more nostalgic than normal:

"Thank You, God, for helping Avery to get to where he is today. Although I'd never want to live through the past few months again, I'm forever humbled by the experience. I feel so fortunate—which I'm sure would sound ludicrous to most. I guess it's true that no one can really understand how someone feels unless they've 'walked a mile in their shoes.' I've seen a lot of babies die. Avery is still here, so how could I not feel lucky?

"We have all come so far on this journey, especially Avery. I can't believe the overwhelming love I have for this little guy, so please don't take him from me. Please give the doctors the wisdom to make the right decisions, and give Dr. LeBlanc a steady hand while he's operating on Avery's little heart.

"Please help Jesse to understand why we have virtually deserted her these past few months. Keep her from harm. Wrap Your arms around her and give her the love that we can't right now.

"My mom has been through so much lately. She is a strong woman, stronger than I could have ever thought possible. Yet, she needs You more than ever. Please continue to provide her with this incredible strength.

"Thank You for giving Cam and I the wonderful love to endure these trying times and to provide such amazing support for each other. Help us to keep the faith, and our sanity.

"Please bless all the babies who are fighting for their lives, and provide their families with the strength to come through such traumatic and tragic times.

"In Jesus' name I ask it all. Amen."

Chapter 20
Never A Dull Moment

August 26

Today Avery isn't eating well. He'll try to suck then begin to cry. I don't understand. Yesterday he was eating like a machine. Maybe my milk supply has finally turned into the Sahara Desert. Frankly, I'm surprised that it has lasted this long. So I pump from the rented machine to see if what I suspect has in fact happened. Surprisingly, there's no problem: I fill a bottle in no time. So what's up? Avery can't afford to lose another ounce. My only job is to get him fat, and failing him is not an option.

This continues throughout the day. I even try giving him a bottle, but to no avail. He won't settle and is screaming feverishly. In tears, I phone Dr. Human's office and tell June (his secretary) my situation. She agrees to page Dr. Human immediately and have him call me. Within minutes he calls and I explain what's happening. "Bring him back to the hospital right now and we'll run some tests. I'll wait for you in cardiology," he says in his serious tone.

This is crazy! I haven't even unpacked from our last return. Mechanically, I take the dirty clothes out from the suitcase and add some clean ones. I'm not even sure what I'm putting in, but at this point I don't really care.

"I can't believe this is happening," I repeatedly say to Cam as we endure another two-hour drive back to the hospital. Avery is screaming inconsolably. I'm worried about him having a heart attack because his face is so red, and his heart is racing.

When we pull into the parking lot of the hospital, Cam drops me off at the door before he parks. As Dr. Human promised, he's waiting for us. As soon as I walk into his office and look into his wide, compassionate eyes, I burst into tears. He gently squeezes my shoulder and takes Avery from my arms. He recalls his nickname and softly asks, "Little Monkey Man, what are you up to now?"

Cam arrives just as Dr. Human begins his checkup on Avery. On the surface he can't find anything wrong. He suggests the problem could be an irritation or infection in his throat from all the tubes coming in and out. However, he adds that we won't know anything concrete until we're able to run some more tests tomorrow. Dr. Human realizes that Avery is probably most upset because he is starving, so he arranges a room for us on 3G and sends us to ICU for a nurse to insert an NG feeding tube.

I'm nervous because it is a tricky process. This is how the nurses feed him in ICU when he's on life support. Every three hours we'll have to slowly pour a few ounces of my expressed milk through a funnel connected to the tube going in his nose to his stomach. If Avery receives too much milk or is fed too fast, he'll vomit it all up. Plus, every time before a feeding we need to aspirate his stomach contents with a syringe attached to his tube and test the ph level to make sure the tube hasn't dislodged from his stomach and into his lungs. If this was to happen and we didn't test for it, Avery's lungs would flood and cause him to drown.

Following the insertion of the tube we head towards the dreaded third floor. I haven't been there since Avery's Code Blue because Dr. LeBlanc had let us stay in ICU until we were discharged. The memories of the hall where all the nurses and doctors had run past me to Avery's bed are still vivid. Thoughts of that dreadful day overcome my senses and I become weak in the knees.

Once we get Avery into his bed, we quickly feed him through the NG tube. Finally, content with his belly full of milk, he falls asleep the moment he lays in his crib. I am beyond exhausted, and it won't be long before I'm asleep in my little cot beside his bed. Just as in our last visit to this ward, Cam sets up his makeshift bed with some of the other fathers in the children's playroom.

August 26

Dr. Human comes to our room around 8:00 a.m. Avery and I have been so sleep-deprived we're still sleeping when he arrives. I look a wreck, although I don't really care. Well, that's a lie; it does bother me a little. Dr. Human always looks so distinguished and well-groomed. Here I am wearing an oversized T-shirt, hair standing on end, drool escaping from the side of my mouth, and bed sheet marks on the side of my face. Lovely. Just how I want to appear in front of my hero.

Dr. Human wants to know how Avery fared during the night, so I tell him that he had a good night, waking up twice for an NG feeding. After he finishes taking his vitals, and before he leaves, he asks us to meet him at the echo cardiogram room at 10:00 a.m. I quickly get dressed and run a comb through my hair. It's not much of an improvement, but it will have to do. As I'm about to go tell

Cam, he walks in from the playroom/sleeping quarters looking about as wonderful as me.

At 10:00 a.m. sharp we enter the echo room, and the technician is waiting for us. Echoes are stressful, not because they're invasive, but because Avery needs to stay perfectly still for close to twenty minutes while the hand-held wand moves all around his chest to search for any discrepancies with his heart. Fortunately, Avery is cooperative this time. I'm sure the technician is amused by our singing attempts to keep Avery quiet and still.

Next we are sent to another room where sticky circles attached to wires are placed all over Avery's chest and back. This is an ECG, which tests for irregular heart rhythms. Avery does great. He must be getting used to all this probing and prodding by now. But wow, does he ever scream when they take off the sticky circles.

We haven't waited long in Dr. Human's office when he enters looking a little perplexed and carrying Avery's results in hand. He says, "All the tests look normal, so it's a bit of a guessing game as to what may be the problem. I'm going to test for yeast in his throat. The steroids Avery had once been on have been known occasionally to cause thrush in the throat. If this is the case, it'll be uncomfortable for him to swallow."

Although this isn't a definitive answer, I feel relief. For once we have a potentially non-life threatening diagnosis. After swabbing Avery's mouth, Dr. Human tells us he'll let us know the results as soon as possible.

It's a lovely sunny day, so we have a picnic lunch on the grass outside the hospital. It's odd because we aren't used to being at the hospital and having Avery with us outside. It's so much nicer, but I'd rather be eating lunch with him in our own yard, and alongside Jesse.

After lunch, Cam and Avery head back to our room for a nap. On my way I decide to go visit Bonnie in ICU and find out how Avery's bed buddies are making out. I know Bonnie has just started her first of a four-day rotation. Under the circumstances, she's happy to see me. "What the heck is going on with Little Monkey Man now?" she asks. With a slight grin I reply, "I guess he missed this place."

The little boy Taylor, who has the same heart defect as Avery, is still the same. Although I've been through hell, I still can't comprehend what Taylor and his family must be going through. I know they've been blessed by three great years with him at home, but it's just not enough—not even close. Children are supposed to outlive their parents.

Noah also appears to be about the same. I want to go and talk to his mom while she sits there alone with her hand reaching into Noah's crib rubbing his head. Yet I hold back. How receptive would she be to me? Our sons have the same defects only mine is doing much better. Why am I feeling this way? Could it be survivors' guilt that I've heard about? Slowly I walk towards her, and when she sees me approaching, she gives a quiet smile. She asks how Avery is doing, then begins to fill me in on Noah's condition. She explains that he isn't stable enough to survive the heart surgery he needs. While she speaks, my eyes began to well up.

Oh no, I can't let this happen. She's trying so hard to be strong, and I can't weaken her with my tears. I manage to hold it together long enough to give her a hug and say, "God bless you."

I can't stand to be in ICU another minute. On my way out, I bump into Lisa and Ben in the hallway and have a brief chat with them. Things are still up and down with Tina. She's still very weak and not ready to come off life support yet. Still, Lisa and Ben appear to be in good spirits. I know why: they have hope, which is a lot more than they had a few weeks ago.

This gets me to thinking that if a person who has a healthy child came into ICU they'd think us parents are crazy. How could we be laughing and conversing as our children lay in beds on life support fighting for their lives? I'm sure that's what I would have thought.

My life lessons pertaining to humans' resiliency continues. As long as there's hope, there's the will and spirit to carry on. Equally as important, I've learned to never judge a person until I've walked a mile in their shoes. In Avery's short time with us, he has already taught me some of life's most valuable lessons.

Cam and Avery are still sleeping when I get back to the room, so for a bit, I sit and watch them peacefully sleep. They're awakened when our new roommate checks in, an eight-year-old boy from Merritt named Eddy. Earlier, during his admission, I'd met his mom and received some information about his condition. Eddy was born with a hole in his heart requiring immediate surgery. The surgery was successful. However, now, eight years later, he has returned to Children's Hospital because of an infection in his heart. He'll be having surgery next week. Eddy seems like a really nice boy, small in stature with large eyes the color of coal.

Meeting Eddy makes me wonder if my life will ever be normal or without fear again. Will I have to worry for the rest of my life? If Avery makes it through the next surgery will I still have to worry about heart infections? I feel my blood pressure rise and the throes of an all-out panic attack emerge, but I'm able to stop myself by taking some deep breaths and telling myself: *One day at a time, Kim. Don't get ahead of yourself. Just take one day at a time.* I repeat it in my head over and over again.

Early evening has come, and we get some good news. Tests prove Dr. Human's assessment is correct: Avery merely has thrush in his throat. The nurse immediately begins the antibiotic treatment. Dr. Human comes by a little later to let us know that by tomorrow Avery will probably be feeling much better, and able to nurse again. He also says that with any luck we will be able to go home in a few days. He wants to wait and see that Avery is eating enough and gaining weight. I chuckle to myself when he says, "with any luck," because on one hand I feel our situation is anything but lucky. Yet, on the other hand I feel like I'm the luckiest person in the world because Avery is still here with us.

August 28

Avery is nursing without any challenges so the nurse takes out his NG tube today. It's good news to be able to give my mom on her birthday today. I wish I could be there to celebrate it with her. I feel bad for her because this must be her worst birthday ever, and the first one in nearly forty years without Dad. When I phone her, however, she seems chipper and is excited to hear we'll be back home in the next day or two.

Chapter 21
Am I Living Groundhog Day?

September 1

Yay! We arrive home again. I hope this will be the last time packing and unpacking for a while—at least until we go back to the hospital for Avery's heart catheterization at the end of this month.

Again, being home is bittersweet because our family isn't complete with Jesse not here. The only thing more painful than not seeing her is talking on the phone to her. Whenever we talk all she says is, "Mommy, come home. Please come home." I can't bear it any more; in her eyes I have deserted her, and how can I blame her for feeling this way? I decide it's best to hold off any communication until the day I'm able to bring her home. It's not what my heart wants but it's what my head says is best for her.

I hope I'm making the right decision, but I'll never have an answer. Our last visit was way too difficult for Jesse, and it'd be unjust to repeat it. Fortunately, it's just shy of a week until the chicken pox restraint is up. All I can do is try to be patient and daydream of soon having the rest of the month together with both my children.

In spite of the circumstances, the past couple of days have gone fairly smoothly. I'm still a little nervous having Avery at home without the nurses and doctors at arm's reach. However, the visits from the health nurse and Bonnie provide some reassurance.

Visits from Mom, Steven, and Tammy make the days go by quite quickly. Plus, some of my other friends, Heather, Rhonda, and Tracee come over from time to time to see how we're faring. I notice they look at me differently. I can't describe it, other than to say they gaze at me the way they would at a wounded deer—a mixture of pity and compassion. I know this isn't their intent, and they all mention how much they admire my strength and ability to remain positive.

I particularly enjoy my visit with Rhonda today. She's one of my only close friends who know the pain of losing a parent. She lost her dad a few years ago from a brain aneurysm. Her company brings a comfort to me, probably because we can relate to what it feels like to suddenly lose our fathers.

I love my family and friends, and one day I'll let them know that their love and support has helped me in so many ways. I just wish my Grandma and Dad were here so I could tell them how blessed and fortunate I am to have had their incredible influence in my life. Even though I'm not able to tell them in person, I have a feeling they know.

Once again, my days of trying to live a semi-normal life come to an end. Why am I even surprised? For some reason, Avery stops nursing again! Only this time he nurses for about thirty seconds, then starts to make a strange gulping noise then breaks out in uncontrollable painful screaming. He does the same when I give him a bottle. When the public health nurse comes and weighs him today, she says he has lost fifty grams.

After a call to Dr. Human, we're on our way back to the hospital—once again! I am *so* frustrated. I can't do twelve steps forward then six back anymore. I'm trying to be strong, but the constant setbacks are wearing me out. Although Cam is visibly stressed, he remains a pillar of strength for me, and continues to reassure me everything will be okay. His words of encouragement help me immensely.

We arrive at the hospital about 10:30 p.m. Avery has a bed waiting for him, and following Dr. Human's instructions, the nurse quickly inserts the NG tube and within minutes Avery has a full belly and falls asleep. I can't believe we're back on the dreaded third floor again. What can possibly be the problem this time?

I think for sure I'll fall asleep immediately from sheer exhaustion, but I don't. It feels like two lions are fighting in my stomach. I fear I'm growing weaker by the day, and my optimism is being tested to its limits. Just as I descend one hill, another appears and then another.

Déjà vu. First thing in the morning Dr. Human comes to see us, displaying the same puzzled look as last time. I explain the gulping episodes but he doesn't understand my explanation very well, so he wants me to nurse in front of him and the lactation specialist so they can observe these episodes. I'm horrified! Haven't I already been humbled enough? Now the doctor that I look up to so much, the same doctor who has become my hero, has to see my breasts in action. Yuk! I think: *I had better be able to laugh at this one day.*

At around 11:00 a.m. Avery starts to get hungry so we page Dr. Human. He and another doctor come within minutes. Feeling completely humiliated, I bring Avery to my chest and begin to breastfeed him while they watch closely. Wouldn't you know it! He feeds for ten minutes without any challenges while the doctors watch to see these gulping episodes I've described. Just great! Now they're going to have to come back and watch the *next* feeding.

For the next few hours I wait, riddled with anxiety about the next breastfeeding display. Oh well, it can't be much worse than the first time. He's already seen my breasts once. What's one more time? I'm surprised that the stress hasn't caused my milk supply to disappear completely. *What if Avery feeds great without any problem again? Will Dr. Human think I've finally gone off the deep end and am making things up? What an exercise in humility this is!*

Fortunately, during the next feeding Avery manages to perform for us and exhibit the gulping episodes for the doctors. What a relief! Dr. Human thinks he may know what the problem is. He believes Avery could have a digestive condition called reflux. He says this is a relatively rare condition which can occur following the disruption of many intubations and extubations. So now we have to stay a couple more days to make sure the new medication works. In the meantime, I'll try to breastfeed Avery, and if needed, alternate with NG feeding.

Avery is feeding much better. The medication for reflux appears to be working well, and it looks like we'll be able to go home soon. Dr. Human wants us to wait at least one more day. In his words: "You never know what this Little Monkey Man is capable of doing. He's fooled us many times before." He's right, and it reminds me when Bonnie told me that Avery would be one for the history books at Children's Hospital. She has mentioned many times that she just can't believe his resiliency.

It melts my heart to see Avery so happy and content. I just want to freeze-frame these moments because they've been so far and few between. When he smiles at me, I temporarily forgot all the pain and heartache I have endured the past few months.

I'm passing the time with Bonnie on her breaks, and chatting with some of the parents here. Today Nikcole comes for a visit. If a person could find one friend like Nikcole in a lifetime, I'd consider them very fortunate. I laugh out loud when she gives me heck for not calling her every day with the rundown of events.

Dr. LeBlanc comes up every once in a while to see us and check on Avery. He's happy with what he sees. Today as he's about to leave, he gives us a compassionate look, shakes his head and says, "You poor people. You have had to go through so much." Cam and I look at each other in surprise. This gruff, matter-of-fact man of few words is showing us a warmer, compassionate side. I knew it must have been there somewhere. After all, a person who saves babies' lives every day must possess a special kind of sensitivity.

I run into Eddy's mom today at the cafeteria. I hadn't seen them on the third floor upon our return, and wondered if they'd gone home already. Well, it was anything but that. His mom explains that the morning before his surgery, a piece of the infection in his heart broke off and traveled to his head, leaving him permanently blind in his left eye. Emergency surgery was set up immediately to replace his infected heart valve and remove the infection. It was pretty much touch and go for a while, and he almost died. Fortunately, everything went well, but he'll be in ICU for a few more days.

As she tells me her story, I can't help but stand there with my mouth open. I know all too well her pain, but I also knew the gratitude she feels. Eddy has lost his sight in one eye, but he's alive and here for his family to hold and love.

I'm not sure if most people understand it when I say I'm grateful. Many of my friends and family think life has been unkind to us. Well, yes, to a point. I certainly wouldn't have signed up for a year like this. But I know that if we get to take Avery home healthy, I'll be the happiest, most grateful mom in the world.

Chapter 22
Together Again

September 9

Today is one of the best days I've had in a very long time. This morning Dr. Human comes to our room to confirm Avery's discharge. He feels confident Avery is ready to come home for a few weeks and "fatten up." He's slightly less than eight pounds now, and Dr. Human would like to see him closer to nine pounds.

The next piece of good news is that Jesse has finished her incubation period for chicken pox and can finally come home with us! She never did contract chicken pox even after being directly exposed to it, so she could've been with us all along. Oh well, it's over now and it's better to be safe than sorry. Now we can focus on spending some quality time together. I'm bursting at the seams to think our family will be together at home for three whole weeks. For some, three weeks may not seem like much, but at this point, I'll take any morsel of normalcy I can get!

I'm thrilled we've made it to this point, yet the stress of Avery's soon—and biggest—surgery looms in my thoughts. I determine I won't let this dampen our time together and I'll put into practice one of the valuable life lessons Grandma taught me: "Appreciate each day because tomorrow isn't promised to anyone."

It's another beautiful sunny day as we pull into the driveway. Mom and Jesse are anxiously waiting at our house. Jesse is outside playing in the sand box and hasn't noticed us arrive. I startle her when I call out her name. With her hair all messy and dried purple Popsicle on her cheeks, she looks more beautiful then ever. She throws her hands in the air and kicks a flurry of sand as she begins to run towards us at mach one speed. Jesse doesn't even slow down when she leaps on me, straddling her legs around my waist. Cam and Avery are right behind me and we all join in on a big group hug. Our family is complete again, and that is all that matters in my world right now.

Jesse can't stop staring at Avery, probably wondering if this is the same little guy she's seen hooked up to so many machines. Stroking his head in delight, she repeats several times, "This Avery. This Avery." Then she points to the sky and says, "Grandpa up sky." I think she's introducing Avery to Grandpa. She wants to include him in this celebration too.

I fight back the tears in this bittersweet moment. "Yes, Jesse. Grandpa is watching us from heaven, and he's so happy we're all together again."

Chapter 23
A New Kind of Normal

September 28

Several weeks have passed since my last entry. I've been so preoccupied with spending every minute possible with Avery and Jesse, relishing this temporary reprieve. It's been the best time ever, and a sense of normalcy has returned—only the definition of "normal" has changed greatly for me. I have never equated normal as being associated with "blessed."

So far, Avery has been feeling terrific and nursing wonderfully. Faith, the nurse from our local hospital, comes every second day to weigh Avery and to check his vitals. She's amazed at his progress, especially his weight gain: he's close to nine pounds. I'm not surprised; every time I turn around Avery wants to eat. Nine pounds is the magic number Dr. Human wants him to be for the open heart surgery.

This reminds me of our pre-admissions appointment with Dr. LeBlanc in a few days, to see if Avery is ready for the tentative October 1 surgery date. For most of this time at home, I've been able to keep the thought of Avery's next surgery at bay. I know it's silly, but I daydream we'll go to the hospital only to find that Avery has been miraculously cured. He looks so healthy now. His skin has gone from gray/blue to more of a slight rosy hue. It is hard to believe he needs this next heart surgery to survive.

Jesse is doing amazingly well too. She has started preschool, and is adjusting fine. However, she has a meltdown every time I try to leave. When I drop her off I tell her, "I'll be back in a couple of hours," but considering how many times I've left her for indefinite periods of time, I can't blame her for getting upset. Her world has been turned upside down and words are of no comfort. After all she's been through she probably wonders if I'm coming back again. It's very emotional dropping her off.

Picking her up after school almost makes the ordeal worthwhile. It's the most welcoming reception one could ever hope to receive. I feel like I'm the most special mom in the world as she runs and jumps into my arms every time I pick her up. I notice many of the other children's lack of enthusiasm to see their parents, and how their moms smile as they watch our reunions.

So far our time home has gone smoothly except for a few stressful moments. Most are fleeting, like when Avery's face went all red and I thought he was about to have a heart attack—only to find out he was just struggling to push out a big bowel movement. Or when Jesse thought she could pick him up and put him on the swing.

Cam has gone back to work. He didn't have much of a choice. We're flat broke and really don't want to borrow any more money from our parents. Having no income for the past four months has really taken a toll. Frankly, I don't care if we even own a house anymore, but in reality it is a good idea to be able to provide a roof over our children's heads. It's difficult for Cam to leave us though. He calls me about six times a day to see how we're doing.

Mom comes over every day to watch Avery while I take her truck to drop Jesse off at preschool. We can't afford insurance on both our vehicles, so this is a practical solution. Mom doesn't mind at all. The first few times it was a little scary for her to be alone with Avery, but after a couple days she was better with it. Fortunately, Jesse's school is only ten minutes away, so I'm not gone long.

I think the daily visits are helpful for Mom. She seems to be coping without Dad as well as can be expected, and I'm so proud of her. She had spent over forty years with Dad, yet, already she's carrying on and taking on all Dad's chores without complaint. Quite often when she talks about him, or when she tells a story about the two of them, she uses the present tense as though he's still here. I know she misses him like crazy, and so do I. Dad is in my thoughts at least a hundred times a day. I still can't believe he's gone.

I just can't lose Avery too.

Steven appears to be moving along okay. He and Tammy come to visit quite often, plus we see him at Mom's every Sunday for dinner. He's been much quieter since Dad died. The two of them were extremely close, never a day passing without them seeing each other.

Tracee has kindly given me a few checks from the profit of our business, which helps our financial woes a little. I can't imagine leaving Avery and going back to work after he comes home from the hospital. I can't think about that now. Besides, Tracee said she and Nordina are working well as a team.

The house is often full of visitors. A couple days after we first arrived home, Nikcole and Macky came over with a beautiful card. When I opened it I almost fell off my chair. Inside was a check for four hundred dollars and a bunch of pictures. A group of our friends had got together and had a big garage sale to raise money for us. The pictures were of everyone helping out. The funniest picture was of our friend, Herb, dressed up in some of the women's clothes that were for sale, harassing the shoppers to buy things.

I most enjoy the visits from Bonnie. She visits often on her days off and stays overnight. She keeps asking if she's wearing out her welcome, and my reply always is, "Come as often as you want. You can even move in." She told me the other day that she's canceling the holidays she had booked for October, so she can take care of Avery after his open heart surgery. The bond between them continues to amaze me. Avery has his own Florence Nightingale.

Chapter 24

The Calm Before The Storm

September 30

Today Avery is four months old. Reflecting on these months is bittersweet. In many ways they have been the worst time of my life, but there are moments where I feel blessed. Avery is a miracle, and our lives are extra-special because of him.

Today is pre-admission at Children's Hospital. We have an appointment with Dr. LeBlanc and Dr. Human to discuss the surgery. Once again the butterflies in my stomach furiously flutter as we make the trip to Vancouver. I feel we're approaching the light at the end of this long dark tunnel, but I'm scared to death. My original request to God was for a little time spent with Avery at home, but now that's not nearly enough. So many parents I met at the hospital didn't even get a week with their baby, and I do feel blessed that I have had four months, but I must have much more.

After taking Jesse to Cam's parents, we hit the road about 8:00 a.m. Leaving Jesse is as agonizing as ever. She's just getting used to a little normalcy, and now it's ruined again. Since May, I have come and gone so many times, will she ever be able to trust me to be a stable person in her life?

During the drive, I distract myself with mindless thoughts. I wonder if Dr. LeBlanc and Dr. Human will notice how different Cam and I look without the sleep-deprived dark circles around our eyes, messy hair, and dirty wrinkled clothes. Three and a half weeks at home has made a big difference. During our hospital hiatus I have actually began to care a little about how I look again. I have gotten so used to not wearing makeup that when I put some on I laughed at how funny it looked.

Once we arrive, we head straight for cardiology. A nurse weighs Avery, and to our delight he is 9.9 pounds. Next he has an X-ray, an ECG, and all this other stuff that has become routine.

Finally, my two heroes arrive and I can tell that they're pleased with what they see. Dr. Human comments on how beneficial the time Avery had at home has been. They're very disappointed to tell us, however, that Avery's surgery has been postponed to October 2. Dr. Human emphatically stated how distressed he is. However, it can't be avoided because there's a backlog of surgeries, and when a critical situation arises, it takes precedence. I understand, and as much as I desire to be one step closer to the end of this nightmare, the delay means I'm guaranteed at least one more day with my son.

Dr. LeBlanc goes through the surgery timeline with us. He says all in one breath, "Surgery will begin at 8:00 a.m., finishing approximately six hours later. Avery's heart will be stopped and the heart and lung machine will keep his organs functioning. Once surgery is completed, Avery's heart will be resuscitated."

The all-too-familiar fear rapidly returns, and his words begin to sound muffled. He continues talking while I watch his lips move, but I've become oblivious to what he's saying.

Tripping over my tongue I ask, "What's the success rate?" It's a question I have always been too afraid to ask. I remember Dr.

Human telling me that the Switch generally has good success, but what does that mean? I also remember there have only been two other premature Transposition babies at Children's Hospital, and neither one made it.

Full of confidence, Dr. LeBlanc replies, "The mortality rate is about eight percent."

"Yes," I say, "but that's with term Transposition babies. The mortality rate for preemies is *one hundred percent*."

He explains this is why they haven't proceeded with the Switch right away. This is also why, when Avery arrived at the hospital, they made phone calls all over North America to find the best course of action. From the information they gathered, they decided to do the other heart surgeries first, in order to prep and strengthen Avery's heart, buying more time for him to grow. Dr. LeBlanc also adds that Avery is currently the size of a healthy term baby, so being underweight is no longer an issue.

The answer provides little comfort. Eight percent mortality is okay odds, but I also know how shaky Avery's track record is from his other even less complicated surgeries. Once our meeting is over, we thank both doctors and go on our way. There's nothing left to say. It's in God's hands now.

On our drive home a melancholy mood sets in while Cam and I attempt to mentally prepare for the next—and hopefully last—hurdle of this crazy journey. We arrive back in Chilliwack to pick up Jesse and my spirits lift once I see her beautiful smile. She looks surprised to see us, perhaps thinking: *Gee, usually when they go, they're gone for weeks.*

When I talk to Bonnie on the phone tonight to tell her the news, she isn't very happy about the date being bumped. She's scheduled to be Avery's nurse on the evening shift the day of his surgery, 7:00

p.m. to 7:00 a.m. the following day. Her plan was to hang out with us Thursday, the day of the surgery then be Avery's nurse that evening. Now she has to try to switch her shift to Friday night.

Chapter 25
The Time Has Come

October 2

I took Jesse to Mom's last night because we had to leave at 5:00 this morning. Once again, we endured the heartbreaking task of saying goodbye. Jesse snuggled into my chest for a long time, begging me not to leave her. Her pouting glare at our suitcases told me she knew we'd be gone a while. With tears falling down my cheeks, I told her this would be the last time, and we'd be back soon, but my words meant nothing. I knew I just had to turn and walk away as Mom held her back.

Or course I didn't get much sleep last night. I spent most of the night staring at Avery and saying many prayers. My anxious nerves don't allow me to feel tired now though. I feel like I've consumed a gallon of coffee. As we drive to Vancouver, Avery sleeps soundly, unsuspecting that in a few hours his chest will be cut open and his heart will literally be in the hands of Dr. LeBlanc.

To divert my attention from the looming operation, I reflect on some of my earlier experiences at the hospital. I remember a mom saying goodbye to her baby just before he was taken away from ICU for heart surgery. She held his little hand and said, "If it's your time to go to God, I'll understand. I'll be okay." At the time I didn't know quite what to think of that. Part of me thought it was a self-less gesture of great love, but part of me thought she was crazy. I look down at Avery and say, "You don't go anywhere. You stay right here with us. Stay strong and fight as hard as you can." I don't care about being selfless. I just want Avery to live.

We arrive at the hospital shortly after 6:30 a.m., and check into surgery daycare. Bonnie is waiting for us. She hasn't been able to switch her shift, so she had to work all through the night until 7:00 this morning. Yet she insists on staying with us today throughout the surgery. The poor girl hasn't slept since Wednesday night. I tell her I'll totally understand if she were to go home, but she says, "Absolutely no way. I'll get enough sleep when I'm dead."

As we pass the cafeteria, I see Dr. LeBlanc sitting at a table all by himself, drinking a coffee. What must he be thinking? He knows he's going to make us the happiest parents in the world or the saddest. Avery may die under his hand, or he might live. How can he have all that on his shoulders, yet keep a steady hand while he's operating on my son's walnut-sized heart?

Everything this morning feels like it's happening in slow motion. We sit in a little cubicle waiting for the anesthesiologist to come and check Avery's vital signs before surgery. Shortly after 7:00 a.m., Bonnie and Linda come to see us. We all wait together, trying to make small talk to pass the time. About 7:30 a young, handsome anesthesiologist arrives. As he's checking Avery's vital signs, I can't believe what I say. I actually ask, "Is it possible a miracle has occurred and Avery's heart is fixed?"

He turns toward me with a compassionate look. "I'm afraid not."

I don't care if he thinks I'm crazy. After all, miracles do happen, and I'm not about to become a disbeliever now. The fact that Avery is still alive demonstrates the power of miracles.

Shortly after Avery's checkup, Dr. LeBlanc comes by. He looks me straight in the eye and says, "I will take good care of him." Then he looks at Avery and says, "Now you behave today, Avery. No funny business."

I grin nervously and say, "I hope the coffee we saw you drinking this morning was decaf."

He chuckles and as he turns to leave, he says, "I will see you soon."

Shortly before 8:00 a.m., the OR nurse arrives to take Avery. We all take a minute to say our goodbyes. I feel removed from my body, like I'm hovering above watching the whole process take place. I see a very frightened girl handing over her baby to the nurse, every part of her body consumed with helpless despair. My arms extend mechanically and I pass Avery into her arms. Words fail me, and tears fill my eyes. When I turn to get a hug from Cam, I see everyone else crying too.

The long wait begins. I never understood how I was able to endure the other surgery waits. I certainly don't know how I'm going to make it through this one. For the most part, Bonnie, Cam, and I sit outside and talk about mindless things, like all the ICU nurses' love lives, and other gossipy stuff. I can't carry on an intelligent conversation if my life depended on it.

A few times I burst into tears as I imagine Avery lying on the operating table with his chest cut wide open and Dr. LeBlanc's large hands working on his heart. It's almost impossible to keep from thinking these thoughts, but as soon as they enter my mind I visualize Dr. LeBlanc coming to tell us that the surgery was a success, and then me leaping into his arms and knocking him over. I picture Avery celebrating his first birthday with a huge party.

The last couple hours of waiting are the worst. We move into a small waiting room where Dr. LeBlanc will be coming to tell us the news about the surgery. There are no windows, only a couch and a chair. I thumb through a magazine, flipping pages like a speed reader, oblivious to their content. Once in a while Cam and I glance up at each other at the same time, and try to provide a comforting grin, but we can't mask the desperate looks in our eyes. Nothing can ease the torture of our wait.

The expected six hours isn't up yet when I see movement at the door handle, then it swiftly opens. It is Dr. LeBlanc and he displays a stern look on his face. My heart sinks into the pit of my stomach, and my head spins as I jump out of my seat. Something has gone wrong! It has only been slightly over five hours, and surgery is supposed to take at least six. From the time he enters the room until the time he speaks is probably less than two seconds, but it's enough time for me to play out in my head all the many scenarios of what may have gone wrong.

My eyes fixate on his lips, waiting for them to move. Then finally I hear him speak the words, "Surgery went well, we finished in less time than we thought, and everything went better than anticipated." I hold my breath as he continues, "As I always do after open heart surgery, I have left his chest open because of the heart swelling. In about twenty-four hours I will close it. Right now, Avery is being stabilized in ICU, and you will be able to see him in about fifteen minutes." The words come effortlessly from his mouth, like reading an instruction manual.

I stand there paralyzed. I can't speak. It has all come down to this moment and now I'm in a state of shock. My sense of reality has become distorted. So much has overtaken our lives since May that I dare not believe my ears. *Did I hear him right? Or am I in a middle of a breakdown and I just think I'm hearing this?*

This is the best news I've ever heard in my life, but yet much of my fear remains. What will Avery look like when I see him? Will his chest be open with his heart exposed? Part of me wants to cry for joy, but the other half wants to turn and run. The first thing I do is fling my arms in the air and wrap them tightly around Dr. LeBlanc's shoulders. I must say "Thank you" ten times. He humbly grins and says, "I'm glad I was able to help." *Able to help? What an understatement!* He has saved my son's life. How can I ever repay him?

Cam gives Dr. LeBlanc a heartfelt hug as well, and with tears welling in his eyes, thanks him too.

As Dr. LeBlanc is leaving, he turns and smiles. "Avery is fixed. Now you can finally start to get your life back." Can he be right? Get our life back. What a beautiful thought. But how can he be sure Avery doesn't have any more tricks up his sleeve? This is supposedly the last piece of the puzzle, yet after everything that's happened I can't be sure this is it.

Bonnie, Cam, and I all rejoice in a group hug, and then impatiently sit and wait for the okay to see Avery.

On our way to ICU Bonnie reminds us how Avery will look. I'm glad she does because as we approach his bedside I'm taken back. He's all puffy and has way more machines and wires hooked up to him than I have ever seen before. There are pacemaker wires, chest tubes for drainage, life support tubes, kidney dialysis, IVs, and central lines all over him. Thank goodness for the large bandage covering his open chest. I can't believe what my eyes are seeing, and even more, I can't believe someone can survive all this.

We aren't allowed to get too close right away. So much commotion is surrounding Avery's bed, and for a moment I think something terrible has happened. Bells and whistles are constantly going off, and doctors and nurses are hovering all around him.

I'm standing there, watching them work to try to stabilize Avery when I see Dr. Human look in our direction. He gives us a smile along with a 'thumbs up.' Everything must be okay. In the midst of giving instructions to the doctors and nurses, he pauses to come tell us Avery is doing great.

As we wait for the okay to come to the bedside, I take a moment to look around the familiar surroundings of ICU. I catch a glimpse of Lisa and Ben at Tina's bedside. Wow. After all this time they're still here. Lisa notices me looking in their direction, so they both walk over and give us a hug. We let them know what's going on and ask how Tina is doing. They proceed to tell us Tina has had a few setbacks, but now is doing better and hopefully getting extubated in the next couple of days.

We stand there for a few seconds in silence before agreeing it will be nothing short of a miracle for both our families to leave the hospital with a happy ending. I let out a chuckle when Lisa says, "I'll be really upset if you guys get out of here before us."

When the crowd clears and we're allowed to go to Avery's bedside, my hand trembles while I stroke his little arm and tell him how proud of him I am. At this moment I realize Avery is the biggest hero of all. The tenacity and strength this little guy has is beyond words. I can't even believe it. I just love him so much. God must have some very important plans for this miracle child of ours.

Dr. Human approaches us and says he's more than impressed with Avery's recovery this far.

"He's stable and already peeing on his own. We're not seeing the same complications we normally have seen following Avery's prior surgeries." I can tell he's delighted, and probably more relieved than anything. He's not displaying the usual disconcerted look that he normally wears when he talks to me. This time his big brown eyes look at me warmly, accompanying a happy smile.

I ask him, "Do you think Avery will remain stable without any 'hiccups'?"

He replies, "I can't say for certain, but probably 'yes' because, as I mentioned before, his heart is finally fixed. So he'll most likely thrive. Avery is working with a normal functioning heart now, and therefore likely won't be experiencing the problems he did before."

I can hardly believe what I'm hearing. I want to scream and do a little dance right here, but I remember where I am. ICU is not typically a place of joy or celebration. There are many anxious people at home waiting for our phone call, so I take a few minutes and run to the pay phone to share the great news. As I make my way there, an exhilarating feeling comes over me. I feel a new lease on life. The tension that has engulfed my body for months is starting to lift.

My fingers can't keep up as I dial my Mom's number. She must have been waiting for our call with one hand on the phone because she answers before the first ring is complete. An anxious voice says, "Hello."

In a rapid ramble I tell her, "Surgery went well and Avery is recovering in ICU." As I say those words, a release of emotions surges through my body, and I begin to cry uncontrollably. For the first time in months I feel the possibility of an end to this nightmare. After we spend the next few minutes on the phone, both bawling, I ask Mom to phone everyone and tell them the great news. Maybe Dr. LeBlanc is right: just maybe we will be able get our lives back.

I quickly make my way back to ICU, crying and smiling all at the same time, wondering if this is all just a dream. Upon my return, Cam takes the opportunity to go call his parents and tell them the news himself.

By now it's been a few days since Bonnie has had any sleep, and her blood shot eyes and dark circles tell me it's starting to catch up to her. I let her know she should go home and get some much-needed rest. I thank her profusely for all her support, and tell her we couldn't have gotten through all this without her. She hugs me and assures me I'm much stronger than I know, and besides Avery, there isn't anyone she is more proud of.

Her kind words make me cry. In some ways I think I *have* been strong throughout this whole ordeal, but in other ways I think I should win the prize for biggest wimp. Oh well, it's irrelevant now. Avery's fate is the only thing that matters.

Throughout the day and into the evening, the doctors are constantly in and out, checking on Avery's progress, displaying their pleasure with what they see. Incredible, Avery is doing fantastic, and I keep pinching myself to ensure I'm in reality. Mrs. Johnston's message reels through my mind: *God told me that Avery will have some very turbulent times, but he will come through them all and live to be strong and healthy.* I also remember the symbols of my Grandma's presence, the four-leaf clovers. They knew all along that Avery would make it.

All that night, and following into the wee hours of the morning, Cam and I stay at Avery's bedside staring at our little miracle, and allowing the enormity of the day's events to sink in. Something feels different than all the other days we've been here. Even though Avery is less than twenty-four hours out of surgery, and not technically "out of the woods," a feeling of comfort is replacing the all-too-familiar despair that has nipped at our heels for many months.

Linda is Avery's nurse this night, and she also says she has a really good feeling about his recovery. She says that when a baby is this stable so soon after surgery, it's usually a good sign.

I notice tonight Noah is still in ICU, so I ask Linda if he has had surgery yet. A sad expression fills her face and she replies that the doctors don't think he is ever going to get strong enough to undergo surgery. I didn't know what to say. It's almost like feeling good makes me feel guilty. I'm so happy that Avery is doing well, but so sad that Noah (who shares the same defect) is not. It's difficult to make sense of it. I'm way too emotional to go to his bedside, and even if I manage to do so, I wouldn't have a clue what to say.

Cam and I keep dozing off at Avery's bedside. I'm quite comfortable in the rocking chair, but Cam keeps falling off his stool, so finally at about 3:00 a.m., Linda practically forces us to go and get a few hours rest. Reluctantly we comply. It has been one of the longest days of our lives, and, I must admit, both of us need a few hours of sound sleep.

October 2 has been a very good day. I can hardly believe my little baby is fixed. Can this really be happening? Can the nightmare finally be ending?

Chapter 26
A Light At The End Of The Tunnel?

October 3

We're dead to the world for a few hours, and when we awake we rush back to ICU still wearing the wrinkly clothes we slept in. When I see Avery, I immediately notice how much his puffiness has gone down, and how good his color is. He is pinker than he has ever been, just like a normal baby. I'm cautiously optimistic, but still feel the need to prepare for the hiccups Avery usually provides us after his surgeries.

Fortunately, the day goes smoothly and we're even able to eat a home-cooked dinner that Lisa has prepared for us. She and Ben live a few minutes from the hospital, which is a nice convenience for them. The homemade lasagna is a welcome treat, and sure beats the cafeteria food. We're very grateful for their kindness.

As always, I have been phoning everyone at home and giving them updates. I tell them to hold off on visiting us until we're out of ICU. Only two people can visit in ICU because there simply isn't the space, plus it's not the best environment for visiting. I would have loved more than anything to see Jesse here, but the pain of departing would be too unfair to her.

Every day brings us a little closer to getting Avery home for good. When we return home and regain some semblance of normalcy again, I wonder how life will have changed for us? It's impossible to go through an experience like this and not be changed. There have been many times in my life I have taken things for granted and overlooked my blessings. My parents and Grandma did provide me with a wonderful sense of appreciation for living, but until a trauma of this magnitude unfolds in a person's own life, I'm not sure if anyone can understand the true measure of gratitude—more importantly, hanging onto it and carrying it with them everyday. My Grandma was able to do that after her accident, and now I believe I will as well.

Chapter 27

Survivors' Guilt Is A Powerful Emotion

October 4

Today starts off very exciting. We come to ICU at around 7:00 a.m., and Mandy is our nurse today. Seeing her bright smile when she says "Good morning!" tells me Avery has had another great night.

For the first time since the open heart surgery I'm able to hold him. Because he still has so many wires and tubes attached to him, it's a very slow and careful process to place him in my arms. I laugh when Cam tells me I'm glowing. Am I finally getting the lovely glow new moms often get? Dr. LeBlanc walks by and when he sees Avery in my arms he slows down. His serious expression changes into a teddy bear smile as he says, "Avery is doing so well that tomorrow may very well be extubation day." Then he continues on his way.

I am shocked to hear those words so soon, and have to double-check with Cam to make sure I heard correctly. Cam said, "Yes, you heard what I heard." Dr. Human was right when he said he suspected Avery will do well because his heart is finally fixed.

I'm embracing the feeling, looking down at Avery in my arms with a permanent grin on my face, when I see Noah's mom,

Bravery | 159

Amanda, walking toward us looking very upset and carrying a big helium balloon in her hand. Without speaking, she walks up to Avery's crib and begins to tie Noah's "Get well" balloon onto the spindle. Immediately I realize what must have happened. But Amanda doesn't say a word, and I don't have a clue what to say. The silence is painful while I watch her fumble to tie the balloon string. I look over at Cam and Mandy for help, but their expressions are vacant like mine. After what seems to be many minutes, but probably not even one, I manage to stutter, "A-Are ... are things ... not well?"

With tears falling from her cheeks, Amanda turns and meekly replies, "Noah passed away last night."

Her words feel like a knife to my chest. All I can say is, "Oh my God. I am so sorry. Is there anything we can do?"

After a long pause, staring at the floor, she slowly shakes her head and whispers, "I guess he just wasn't strong enough. God bless Avery and your family." Then she slowly turns and walks away.

When I turn to Cam and Mandy I see the tears begin to fall. Mandy quickly passes me some tissue so I can stop my tears from falling on Avery who is still cradled in my arms. This is a damn sad day, but Avery is finally doing fabulously. My emotions are all over the place, and I can't describe my feelings. Perhaps I'm experiencing something like survivors' guilt. It hits home how this could have easily been *us*. It could have been me tying Avery's balloon to Noah's crib.

They both had the same defect, but only one lived and the other died. Did God have to pick one or the other? Surely not! But if so, why did He pick Noah to go? Was it because I have prayed more often? Or have I? Could it have been because Dr. Human is a better cardiologist than Noah's doctor? What could it have been? I don't want these silly thoughts to enter my head, but it's difficult to avoid the search for some clarity to these impossible questions.

I can only imagine how Noah's mom must be feeling. Her beautiful baby gave the fight of his life but after a few months lost the battle. He didn't have a chance to know the wonderful person who loved him so much. Amanda didn't have the opportunity to know her son, to watch him grow into a handsome young man—life experiences that so many of us just assume will unfold.

It makes no sense to me why God would bring a life into the world, only to take it as quickly as it enters. What possible purpose can that have, other than to inflict incredible pain onto the loved ones they leave behind? Yes, I knew firsthand how a painful experience can strengthen us, but … not in this situation. Some babies don't even get to open their eyes before they have to go. How can that make anyone stronger? No, it can't. I fail to see any reason, and doubt anyone here on earth has a clue.

So I guess for now I'll add it to my long list of life's conundrums to which I have yet to find an answer. Like my girlfriend Heather says, "There are many questions we have in this lifetime that we won't get any answers to until we meet our Maker."

Chapter 28
Are We There Yet?

October 5

First thing in the morning, Cam and I rush to ICU to await the news about extubation. What a great sight it is to see Bonnie rocking in the chair with a content Avery in her arms. Right away she says with a grin, "I think someone's ready to breathe on his own." I hope she's right, but we must wait for the doctors' morning rounds to confirm Bonnie's notion.

Cam has the hilarious idea of making a little sign that reads, "Please extubate me!" He places it in Avery's tiny hand for the doctors to see upon their rounds. It's impossible to hide our mischievous grins as they approach Avery's bed. They're all wearing their usual concerned looks as they travel from bed to bed checking on each patient. When they reach Avery's space and notice the sign in his hand, grins encroach upon their faces and slight chuckles emerge.

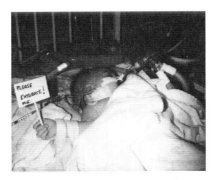
("Please extubate me!")

Cams' sign brings a welcome break from the seriousness, but not the answer we've been hoping for. Dr. Human feels the X-ray of Avery's lungs still looks a little wet, and he wants to be on the safe side and wait another day. It's disappointing, but I'm grateful he's being so cautious.

Nikcole comes for a visit today. I get a lecture because I haven't phoned her with an update for a couple days. She left a message on my cell, but I forgot to phone her back. Of course, she's delighted with Avery's progress, and our positive spirits contribute to a much more enjoyable visit than all the others.

Not much is new with Nikcole except Tracee's car was broken into and her purse stolen. Nikcole said Tracee didn't get too upset because she said it pales in comparison to what we're going through. Avery is already teaching people not to sweat the small stuff. I'm looking forward to learning much more from him. There's a whole new life waiting out there. I can't wait. I'm going to jump in head first.

We spend some of our visit outside, and I notice that autumn has snuck in. The leaves on the trees are changing color and the air is getting crisper. It's hard to believe we've been here for three seasons—spring, summer, and now into fall. It seems so long, but living it every day, it's all been a blur.

Today is our best day yet. The X-rays confirm Avery's lungs are dry and he's ready to come off life support. The tubes come out about 9:00 a.m., and now the fretful wait begins to see if Avery can continue to breathe on his own throughout the day. I'm feeling cautiously optimistic, especially since the doctors are feeling this way as well.

We're lucky to have Lisa bring us dinner again. She's also in an especially chipper mood because Tina is scheduled to be extubated on Friday. It's wonderful to share in each other's excitement. For so long both our families have been battling to make it through each day. Now finally we're able to share an inspiring, hopeful future. Sitting at Avery's beside, it dawns on me how much I'm going to miss everyone here. They've become a tremendous network of support. I want more than anything to get out of this place, but I know I'll miss many people I've come to know throughout the course of this turbulent journey.

Well into the evening Avery is still going strong, and I marvel at the sight of Cam feeding him a bottle. He has a relieved, contented look on his face that I haven't seen for many months. I'm sure that by now we can read each others' thoughts from a simple look. If he can read mine, he knows how lucky I feel to have all his support.

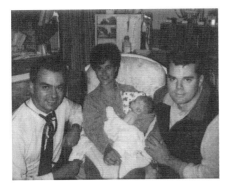
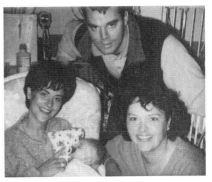

(Dr. Human, me, Avery and Cam)   (Us with nurse Bonnie)

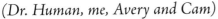

October 7

We say goodbye to ICU—hopefully for the final time—and head to the Observation Ward, the dreaded third floor where the memories are still as fresh as the day of the Code Blue. I remind myself this visit is much different: Avery's heart is fixed now. He still sleeps a lot, but when he's awake he likes to move around, kicking his feet and swinging his arms all over the place, displaying a big grin on his face.

I'm able to nurse Avery today for the first time since surgery and everything goes well. Because he's only at ten pounds in his fifth month, he has a lot of growth to catch up on.

This afternoon Cam takes a trip to the shopping mall to buy Dr. LeBlanc and Dr. Human each a gift, while I stay to write them a letter expressing our gratitude. It's impossible to articulate how thankful we feel, but I do my best. Cam returns with a beautiful designer watch for Dr. LeBlanc and an expensive bottle of wine for Dr. Human. He's had as much difficulty knowing what to get them as I have had preparing the letters. However, no matter what we write them or what we give them, I'm sure our appreciation is apparent.

Although it's Bonnie's day off she comes to the hospital because, in her words, she needs her 'Avery fix.' She's impressed with his progress, and thinks he'll be discharged in a few more days. It's difficult to digest the fact that Avery's days as a patient here are almost over, and his life will begin anew.

Lisa also comes for a visit bringing some good news with her: Tina was extubated today and is breathing strong.

Steven and Tammy come for a visit this evening, and they bring a surprise visitor with them—Tammy's mom, Heather Johnston! As I mentioned, until Avery was born I didn't really know much about Heather, other than she was a very devout Christian. Now I'm in complete awe of this amazing woman. In this short period of time, I feel she has become my guardian angel.

When she walks in behind Tammy and Steven I leap from my chair and almost jump into her arms! She says at the last minute she was able to get off work early to make the trip with Tammy and Steven. It's a pure delight to see her, and even more so to watch the look on her face as she walks over to Avery's crib to hold him for the first time. Her large brown puppy-dog eyes fill with tears as she bends down to give him a kiss on the forehead. I think we all began to cry.

She gently places her finger inside the palm of Avery's hand and in his light slumber he wraps his fingers around hers with a gentle squeeze. Her silent gaze upon Avery lying so peaceful in his crib is a sight I have longed for, a vision that has kept me going through my darkest days. Miraculously, it's here. My prayers have been answered and Heather was right all along.

My expression of heartfelt thanks can't come close to portraying the incredible gratitude I feel for Heather, but that's okay. She knows.

October 9

I'm still pinching myself as more great news keeps coming. Yesterday morning Dr. Human discharges us from Observation to a regular ward. We're lucky to get a private room, and there's even enough room for two cots for both Cam and I. Avery is sleeping much less already, and loves being carried around the room. Walks around the hospital in the stroller are his favorite. He gets a little perturbed when we put him in his crib. I can't blame him, since most of his life has been spent lying in bed, but he does need to keep up on his sleep.

Cam's parents, Madge and Steve, come for a visit today. They are visibly proud grandparents beaming with excitement about Avery's development. Cam shines with joy as he watches them take turns holding Avery.

The biggest surprise of all comes this afternoon when Dr. Human arrives at our room with the news that we can go home tomorrow! I know Avery is doing fantastic but it has only been eight days since his surgery. Dr. Human and the other doctors feel Avery is in top health and is ready as he'll ever be to go home.

"Avery's heart is fixed and as good as new," he says. "He's finally behaving like he's supposed to." He must sense a bit of anxiety in my expression because he adds, "We would never let you leave if we had anything to be reluctant about. But don't hesitate to call me, or come back at anytime if you have any concerns at all." His words are comforting, but hopefully we'll only need to return for checkups. He also asks us to phone his office next week to book a follow-up visit in one month.

We say our goodbyes to Dr. Human today because tomorrow is Sunday and he won't be here then. Tears begin to form in Cam's eyes when he passes him our gift. I hug Dr. Human tightly and tell him how much he means to us. Keeping his composure, he puts the letter in his pocket then looks up at us and says, "Thank you. You're a remarkable family. You've been through too much and I'm delighted to see this day finally arrive for you." He gives Avery a rub on the head, telling him to be a good boy then nods farewell.

It's difficult to say goodbye to Dr. Human. I adore him and look up to him with more respect than almost anyone I've ever met in my life. He won't be a part of our lives anymore, and I'll miss him terribly! I wonder if he has any idea of how much he means to parents like us. I know doctors don't typically get emotionally attached to their patients, but I wonder if he'll miss Avery.

After Dr. Human leaves, Cam and I decide to check Dr. LeBlanc's office to see if he's there because he often stops by on Saturdays. We're in luck as he promptly answers the door. He's surprised to see us, and even more surprised when we hand him his gift. He opens up the letter and begins to read it. Slowly, a gentle smile appears on his face and with misty eyes he looks up at us and says, "Thank you so much. As much as we will miss Avery, I am happy to see an end to your days here. Avery is a very special boy, and he is going to bring you much joy."

My eyes well up as I look down at Avery cradled in my arms and say, "He'd better, after all the fuss he's put us through." This brings welcome laughter.

When Dr. LeBlanc opens his gift and sees the watch, he begins to shake his head and in his thick French accent says, "This is too much. I cannot accept this."

I reply, "You saved Avery's life. You're one of the reasons we're bringing him home tomorrow. It makes us happy to be able to give you a gift as part of our thanks and gratitude."

With a sheepish grin he nods and says, "I understand. Thank you. It is beautiful and I will wear it proudly."

No present can possibly convey our monumental gratitude to Doctor Human and Dr. LeBlanc, but I feel it's important to do what we can.

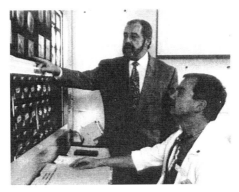

(Dr.Leblanc (standing) with Dr. Human)

Tomorrow is Thanksgiving Day. There isn't anything better in the world to give thanks for than Avery's homecoming. How serendipitous for him to come home on Thanksgiving.

Children's Hospital has been our home, and Avery's entire existence thus far has been under the wings of professional care. We're going to be all on our own now, leaving the entourage of doctors and nurses behind. Now, somehow I'm supposed to go home and raise Avery like any normal baby. I have no clue about what the future should look like anymore, and I'm not the same person I was five months earlier. I'll need to create a new vision board of what life will be like for me. One thing I know is I'll be a different kind of mom because of the new appreciation that's been born in me. My promise was clear: "If I get to bring Avery home healthy, I'll be the happiest mom on earth." My wish has come true, and I can't wait to follow through with my word.

Cam and I decide not to phone and tell anyone the news. The surprise from a phone call saying, "We're home!" will be a much greater Thanksgiving present.

Chapter 29
Walking Papers

October 10

Early this morning the resident doctor comes by with our walking papers. Not a better feeling in the world exists than the one I feel now. We're already packed and ready to go except for one last stop at ICU to say our goodbyes. I had written every one of Avery's nurses a "Thankyou" note and place it in their boxes. Fortunately, Bonnie is working so we're able to say goodbye to her in person. She's already planning to come to our house for a visit on her next day off.

We make our way around ICU, saying goodbye to everyone we know. Lisa starts to cry when she sees us approaching Tina's bed. I know her tears are out of joy for us, but it must be bittersweet because we're going home and they're still waiting. We exchange big hugs and promise to keep in touch. Lisa says that although she wishes it were them, she's delighted to see us go home. Tina is doing excellent and is moving out of ICU today, so I'm sure it won't be long before they'll be going home as well.

Our last stop is at little Taylor's bed. He smiles brightly when we tell him and his parents we're going home. I'm barely able to hold back the tears as Taylor's dad shakes our hands, wishing us good luck. I can understand their difficulty in saying goodbye to us. Taylor has been in Children's' Hospital for longer than Avery, and I know all too well the feeling of seeing another patient go home while you remain. Of course you're happy for them, but you just wish it was you. This time it is us, and I still can't believe it!

Bonnie takes one of her breaks and walks with us to the car. I hurry to the motor home to gather some of our stuff. Cam will come back with his dad in next few days to drive it home. I wait impatiently while Cam takes off all the RV hook-ups and moves the motor home to a storage space. Bonnie knows we're in a mad panic to dash home, so she gives us all a quick hug, and stands there waving until we're out of her sight.

Most of the drive home I anticipate my reunion with Jesse. No more worrying about leaving her, no more being torn apart as I look at her sad face every time we leave her for an indefinite length of time. She won't have to feel we've deserted her anymore.

When we arrive home Avery is very hungry, so as I feed him I phone Mom and say, "Guess where we are?"

"NO way!" she says. "You're not home, are you?"

Just shy of a scream, I reply, "Yes! We've just unloaded our suitcases to make room for Jesse, and we're on our way over as soon as I finish feeding Avery."

I have to hold the phone away from my ear as Mom shrieks in delight.

The usual five-minute drive to Mom's from our house seems twice as long as usual. Jesse gets a surprise of a lifetime when we burst through the door unannounced. She's sitting at the table coloring, and when she turns to see us I think she's going to fall off her chair. She jumps into the air and races over to us with her feet barely touching the ground. She leaps up into my arms and squeezes me tight. The four of us share a big group hug. It's the best hug I've ever had in my life.

I tell Jesse, "We're home for good, together as one happy family."

She points to Avery and with a big smile says, "Let's go. Truck home."

When Mom gives me a welcoming hug I'm overcome with happy emotions. Mom can finally feel some relief knowing her grandson has won his courageous battle. She's been through so much, and yet has remained so strong for me. Elated, she picks up Jesse and dances around the room singing, "Happy times are here again!"

Jesse's strange smile tells me she must be thinking, "What's gotten into you, Grandma?"

For the first time our family is going home to be together. The roller coaster ride is over. Although we bear some wounds that will take a while to heal, and Avery wears a few scars that will forever remind him of his long battle, we stand taller and stronger than ever.

Following our departure from Mom's we decide to drive directly to Cam's parents' house and surprise them with the good news. Jesse is so cute on the drive. She's as bewildered by this day as Cam and me. She keeps looking at me, then Cam, then Avery, then back to me again.

When we arrive at the Gemmell's home, Madge opens the door and looks as though she's about to pass out. She lets out a scream, "You're home!" Although Steve is hard of hearing and in another room at the time, he must have felt the shock waves of her scream. He comes running to the door as though Madge had been attacked. When he sees all of us standing there, he looks as though he's seen a ghost. Enormous grins fill their faces while they take turns holding their grandson.

We return to Mom's house tonight, along with the Gemmell's for the best Thanksgiving meal I will ever have the pleasure of attending. Mom was only planning to have dinner for Steve, Tammy and Jesse but luckily she always cooks for an army, so there was plenty of food. I always knew Thanksgiving Day was meant for giving thanks—I just never realized how much I have to be thankful for.

Chapter 30
A Whole New World

November 14

It's been over a month since we have been home, and until today I haven't had much inclination to write. It's nice to not have to think or focus on anything. I have just wanted to relish the joy of spending time with my family.

We're adjusting smoothly to our new life. I still have my bouts of anxiety every now and again, but I think that is to be expected. I called 911 the other day because Avery was crying for no apparent reason, and wouldn't stop. Cam had already left for work, so I was alone with Jesse and Avery when he started to cry. At least ten minutes passed and Avery's face was getting so red that I feared he might be having a heart attack. It was just awful. I was holding Avery while I was on the phone with the operator trying to explain the situation but he couldn't hear me because of Avery's loud screams. He kept telling me to put the baby down, but I couldn't do it. Finally, after about his fourth attempt he screamed at me, "Put the baby down!" I did, and proceeded to explain what was happening. Mom and Cam arrived simultaneously, both racing down the driveway in a mad panic, only a few minutes prior to the ambulance.

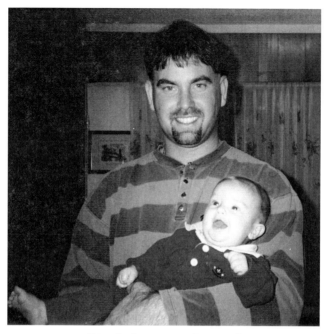

(Uncle Steven and Avery)

By this time, Avery's loud cries had subsided to uncomfortable whimpers. The paramedics checked him out thoroughly but could find nothing wrong. To be on the safe side we took him to our local pediatrician who also could find no evidence of anything being wrong. Fortunately, following the incident, Avery acted totally fine.

Other than that particular challenge, Avery is a happy, thriving baby, and already thirteen pounds. That's still light for being almost six months old, but it's great progress. His development in all other aspects is good too. Shortly after returning home we arranged for a developmental specialist to come and work with Avery twice a week. Dr. Human warned us that Avery's physical and mental development would have some catching up to do because most of his newborn life was spent in bed. A physiotherapist is starting work with him next week to strengthen his muscles. He's already trying to pull himself up.

Jesse is adjusting very well to sharing her home with Avery. She plays with him a lot, sometimes annoying him with all the toys she shakes in front of his face, along with all the kisses she smothers him with. It's funny to watch, especially when Avery sometimes gets ahold of whatever Jesse is shaking in his face. He takes a moment to examine it, then with a big grin tosses it across the room and watches Jesse run to get it. She never seems to tire of trying to find ways to entertain her little brother.

I'm a little concerned about the occasional tantrums Jesse exhibits. I'm sure much of it is caused by all the confusion life bestowed upon her, plus the doctors mentioned her limited vocabulary will cause some frustration until she catches up.

The week following our return home, Cam went back to work. He desperately needed to because we have a lot of financial catching up to do. Tracee tells me everything is going well with the business, and her generosity in writing me a few checks has helped. I feel a little guilty about not being much help to her, yet it's out of my control. I can't leave Avery to go back to work. It's hard enough leaving him for an hour to go get groceries.

The support from friends and family is amazing and gifts are still coming in. A couple of weeks ago some of the employees from Cam's work put on a fundraiser for us. A local pub donated a keg of beer to them with all the profits from the sales going to a fund for us. They raised over four hundred dollars. Cam and I were overcome with gratitude for their generosity.

I see Mom almost every day. On the days Jesse goes to preschool, Mom watches Avery while I borrow her truck to take Jesse to school. (We're trying to cut costs by only having one vehicle on the road.) Although Mom doesn't divulge her full feelings to me, I see in her eyes how much she misses Dad. There is such a huge void in her life now. We don't talk about Dad a lot because we both start to cry, so we try to protect each other from the pain.

I'm crazy with missing Dad. I dream about him all the time, and in my dreams he's always healthy and happy. When we were in the hospital my whole focus was on Avery, so now that we're home, I think about Dad a lot more. I haven't been able to look at the picture of Dad holding Avery yet. I haven't even been able to bring myself to ask Mom if she has developed the film.

Occasionally Jesse points up into the air and says, "Grandpa." A few weeks ago, after she pointed to the sky and said his name, I asked her, "Do you see Grandpa?"

She said, "Yes."

My jaw dropped to the ground. "Does he say anything? Does he talk to you?"

"Yes."

"What does he say?"

With a big grin she said, "Jesse, love you."

Goosebumps rippled up my arms, and I was reminded of the four-leaf clovers sent to me from Grandma. They're both with us, and I know in some capacity Jesse sees him. I don't think three-year-olds know how to lie.

We've been having many visits from friends. Bonnie has already come out a couple times. I love her visits, and the connection we share is so comfortable. She's one of my only friends that can begin to understand who I am now, and what I have gone through. I probably have a greater understanding of her than many of her friends do because I have seen firsthand what she does everyday, and what kind of hero she is.

Bonnie's boyfriend Jack has recently left her, so she is extremely sad. She loves him dearly and is devastated to lose him. She has more time on hers hands now, so we are happy to see more of her.

Today I write in my journal: "I think this might be my last entry. It's time to close you up and put you on the shelf. I'm a little sad to say goodbye, but I feel it's time. I'm surprised I was able to keep you going, especially on the very dark days. I'm very glad I did because I will open you up every now and again when I need a dose of humble pie. I'm sure there are going to be a few of those days. You will always be there to remind me how precious life is, and how quickly the bottom can fall out."

I'm definitely a different person now than I was in the beginning of this journal. My rose-colored glasses may be broken, but my spirit remains strong.

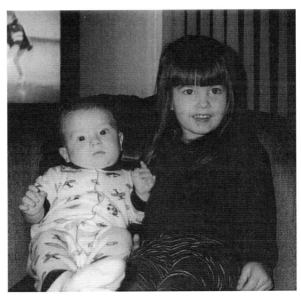

('Home at last' Avery and Jesse)

TO AVERY

I have written this journal for you to read when you get older, so you'll always know how very special you are, and how much you are loved by so many people. You have touched the lives of people you will never even know, and are a hero in many ways. You have already done so much to make this world a better place. You have profoundly affected the hearts of so many people. I am in wonder of your will and strength to survive. So many times we almost lost you, but you defied all odds. You are a miracle and I know God has special plans for you!

I only wish you could have grown up knowing your Grandpa. You weren't quite two months old when he died, but he got to love you a lifetime in that small period. He was so proud of your fight and your spirit. We have one picture of him holding you. Your Grandma took it a few days before he died. I can't wait to show it to you, and tell you all about him. I don't know many people like him who had such a loving, caring heart for his family and friends. Even though he's no longer here, we're lucky because you, Jesse, and I all have a little part of him inside us, so he will always live on through us.

Thank you, Avery, for making your Dad and me the proudest parents in the world. You are my hero. I love you so much!

TO JESSE

Throughout these past months your life was torn apart, yet you have been the best little girl in the world. I can't describe the pain I felt being apart from you all that time. Those months must have been awful for you, especially not knowing why we were leaving you, and whether or when we'd be coming back.

When your Grandpa died, I was so worried about you. He was your best friend in the whole world. The two of you would spend hours together each week. Even if he had lots of work to do, it would be put aside to spend time with you. Every day you would ask to see him at least ten times, or until I put you in the car and drove you there. Leaving was a whole other story. You would scream and cry to stay, so Grandpa would say, "Okay, Jesse, you stay here with me for a while and I'll drive you home later." Then you'd have a big grin from ear to ear. Even though I didn't want you to always get your way, I could never say no to Dad. Now, I'm so glad that I let him spoil you because it gave you more time to spend with him. You loved him more than anyone, and I'll always try and keep those memories alive for you.

Talking about you and him reminds me of a funny story I'd like to share with you. In Grandpa's eyes, you could never do any wrong, and no one was allowed to give you heck when he was around. One day you were at Grandpa and Grandma's house playing with a big bucket of rocks that Grandma had to make some stepping stones. We tried to take the bucket away from you because rocks were flying everywhere through the house, but you had a little fit, so Grandpa said to let you play with the rocks and he'd clean them up later. Well, it probably took him at least three hours because there were a thousand pebbles everywhere. Grandpa didn't care though. As along as you were happy, that was all that mattered to him.

You've been saying "Grandpa" a lot and pointing in the air. When I ask you if you see him you smile and say, "Yes." I know he's here with us, and I'm so happy you can see him. He will be with you, guiding and protecting you forever.

I want to thank you, Jesse, for being the best daughter a mother could ask for. I love you so much.

My Grandma always said, "You're as beautiful outside as you are on the inside." That's you, Jesse. Remind me sometime to tell you about your great-Grandma. She was truly remarkable.

TO MOM

I don't know what I would've done without you, especially this past year. It meant so much to know I could always count on you. I couldn't have made it through as well as I did without your support. I knew there wasn't anything you wouldn't have done for me.

You have helped me become a strong, confident person who will always believe that anything is possible. I often remember my first day of kindergarten when I insisted that I couldn't go in. We were standing in the parking lot as you were trying to coach me into the school. I said, "I can't go in! I can't do it!" You knelt down at my eye level and said with a stern, serious face, "There is no such word as *can't*."

Those words must have had quite an impact because off I went into the school. Whenever I'm reluctant or feeling insecure, I remind myself of that day, and am filled with the same encouragement I felt when you spoke those words to me over twenty-five years ago.

Your unconditional love and support have provided me with all the tools I will ever need to be a great mom, daughter, friend, and wife. I am most lucky and blessed to have you as my mom. Thank you. I'll love you forever.

TO CAM

It's hard to even know where to begin. This year would have torn up and spit out most couples, yet it has united us even more. During our many months in the hospital, and when Dad died, there were so many times I thought I was going to end up a puddle on the floor. Somehow you always caught me before I fell and held me together. I seriously don't know what I would ever do without you. Sometimes I probably come across as an independent old goat, but the truth is, I'm strong because I have you beside me.

I know there are many times we each came so close to a breakdown, but it was our love and support for each other that held us together. Throughout our hospital experience I saw many couples start to pass blame on each other, or just get frustrated with each other because of their situation. I'm amazed that our words always remained positive and supportive. We never lost sight of each other's pain and the desire to ease it.

I'm sure there will be rough patches ahead. All families face them. But I have the faith we will beat any obstacles that come our way. This year demonstrated a newfound respect in our relationship, and I'm confident we can overcome any challenges that come our way.

I wasn't sure if I would be able to find someone who measured up in my Dad's eyes, until I met you. I know he used to worry a lot about who my boyfriends were, or who I would marry. He died knowing I had the best husband, one who would always take good care of me.

Thank you. I'm so proud to be your wife.

Chapter 31
Goodbye 1998

I know I said I wasn't going to add any more entries to my journal. However, when I stumbled across it today I felt compelled. There are a few loose ends I need to address, especially in regards to the little ones we grew to know at the hospital.

Thankfully, 1999 is off to a smooth start. Avery continues to amaze us every day with his steady progress. He's sitting up now and interacting with Jesse a lot more. Right now I'm in the family room watching them play with the toys they received for Christmas. It's a beautiful sight. Jesse continues to be a big help to Avery, patiently retrieving the toys he throws around. She likes to make him laugh by making all kinds of weird, funny faces. Avery is fascinated with how Jesse moves around the room, and wishes he could be mobile like her.

Recently he's getting down on all fours and rocking back and forth, so I know that crawling is just around the corner. With his incredible amount of energy, it's difficult to believe he's had any heart surgeries. He goes nuts in his jolly jumper, bouncing around like a Mexican jumping bean, and screaming "Da, da!" at the top of his lungs.

A couple of days ago Jesse, Avery and I went into Vancouver for a visit at Lisa and Ben's house to see Tina. Yes, Tina made it home after all! Having a visit together outside the hospital was wonderful. Watching the two of them roll around the floor was a miracle. Tina has had some continuing health challenges, however. Despite trying everything, Tina won't eat or drink orally, and needs to be fed a liquid diet through a tube inserted into her abdomen. The doctors said Tina spent so much time being fed nutrients intravenously that she has lost the swallowing reflex that babies are born with. They're uncertain as to if or when she'll ever be able to swallow food normally. It was fun to watch them roll around like typical babies unaware of the adversities they had conquered.

Taylor, the little three-year-old boy who'd had the same heart defect as Avery passed away in December. I learned about little Taylor's fate when Bonnie was over for a visit. She had received a phone call from another ICU nurse with the terrible news. Taylor had been showing some signs of heart distress for some time, and finally his tiny heart went into cardiac arrest and he couldn't be revived. The news devastated Bonnie and I, and we sat in my house and cried all afternoon. I'm most sorry for his passing, but it scares me that Taylor and Noah both had the same defect as Avery, yet they have both died and Avery has lived. Life just doesn't make sense sometimes and it would be a futile attempt to try to understand.

A few days after Taylor's passing, Bonnie and I attended a lovely service for him in the Chapel at Children's Hospital. There wasn't a dry eye to be found as Dr. Human gave a wonderfully touching eulogy. Complete despair and sorrow filled Gord and Cynthia's presence. Their grave faces and mechanical movements were void of emotion. Part of them had died.

After the service Bonnie and I approached them and gave them heartfelt hugs. All I could manage to stutter was, "I ... I am so sorry." I guess there wasn't much more that could be said, other than that sometimes "God's will" is impossible to understand. All they needed to know was they had the heartfelt support from all their loved ones. They thanked us for coming and gave a special thanks to Bonnie for her loving and outstanding care with Taylor. Then they wished me the best of luck for Avery, and a healthy future. Most of my drive home was filled with tears and nostalgic thoughts of the past year.

Recently Bonnie gave me news about Anthony, the little boy who had drowned in the pool. After taking him off life support, his parents moved him to Sunny Hill Rehabilitation Center, but Bonnie heard from a nurse who works there that Anthony hasn't regained any cognitive abilities. The family still prays for a miracle.

I still feel survivors' guilt, but I resolve to remain grateful that Avery is here. We'll never know, at least here on earth, why one lives and another dies.

On a lighter note, tomorrow is going to be Jesse's fourth birthday, and she's very excited about the dinner we'll be having for her together with Mom, Steven, Tammy, Madge, and Steve. I love it when she gets excited about an event. The passion in her eyes ignites a contagious grin.

Jesse's frustration level appears to be improving, and she's enjoying preschool. Although her vocabulary isn't up to speed with her peers, it's encouraging to see some progress.

Everything with Cam is going suitably. He's working hard at his sales job, trying to earn as much money as possible so we can catch up financially. Although the steady paychecks coming in are nice, being away from the kids all day is painful for him. Every day he races home to spend as much time as possible with us. He's a wonderful father, and I couldn't be more proud of him. I finally feel like we're becoming husband and wife again, rather than just a support team, numb to any intimacy.

We sold our house and are preparing to move at the end of this month. We bought a really nice house that, surprisingly, cost a little less than this one—plus our acquired equity will help lessen our debt load. Although I really like this house, I'm not so concerned with where we live anymore as much as the quality of time spent where I live. Of course I want to be able to provide my children with everything wonderful, but good health prevails over any other need.

We're truly blessed to live in a country that provides the best hospitals, along with incredible doctors and nurses. In many parts of the world, Avery would have died because we couldn't have afforded the health care.

I sold my half of *Friend of a Friend* to Tracee. Going back to work is out of the question. There's no doubt it will be a long time before I'm able work outside the home. Our family has been through too much, and we need some healing time. Every day I spend with the kids is so valuable. I decided that I would rather make monetary sacrifices in order to spend the time with Avery and Jesse.

Mom still comes over regularly, and we go to her house every Sunday for dinner. Since Dad passed away, she's slowly getting adjusted to living a new life. She joined a curling club with some of her girlfriends, and is talking about taking up golf in the spring. Bonnie will love that because they can go golfing together when she comes out for visits.

My gratefulness continues constant every day and every once in a while I still feel the need to pinch myself to believe I'm now living this wonderful life with two healthy children. Sometimes I get a little scared when I remember how a happy life can be taken away in a blink of an eye. There's no doubt that the experiences with Avery have left me in a somewhat sensitive state. If I'm away from home without Avery and hear an ambulance, my heart beat races and my blood pressure rapidly rises because I fear they're on their way to our house. I know it sounds silly, and I know the odds are 1 in 70,000 (the number of people living in Chilliwack), but my mind doesn't always think logically in such moments.

People tell me all the time how terrible it was for my dad to die at such a young age, and how I must feel ripped off—but I don't agree at all. Of course I wish I would have had many more years with him. I would have loved him to know Avery, and to have spent more time with Jesse. But no, I don't feel bitter. Dad had a full life, including marrying his soul mate, becoming a successful business owner, living to see his healthy children grow up and get married, and then spending his last years learning to slow down and share precious time with his granddaughter. Little Taylor didn't even have a chance to learn how to ride a bike. His parents will never get the opportunity to watch him grow into a handsome young man. Nor will they be able to watch him graduate, or dance at his wedding. So no, I don't feel cheated at all. I'm lucky. I spent many wonderful years with my dad and have a lifetime of great memories to cherish.

If I could tell people one thing to keep alive in their hearts forever, it would be: love and cherish your children unconditionally every day. And I'd add: memorize each wonderful expression in their face. Praise their accomplishments, because in their eyes we are their heroes—and they are ours. Watch them as they sleep and be enthralled by their presence. Stop what you're doing when they want a minute of your time because tomorrow isn't promised to anyone.

I'm truly blessed for having awakened to embrace these precious life lessons.

It's funny to watch the expression on some people's face when I say I'm a lucky person. They just don't get it. Like the words I live by say, "A person can't begin to understand someone's life until they've walked a mile in their shoes." My shoes may show a lot of wear, and have a lot of scuffs, but I wouldn't trade them in for anything.

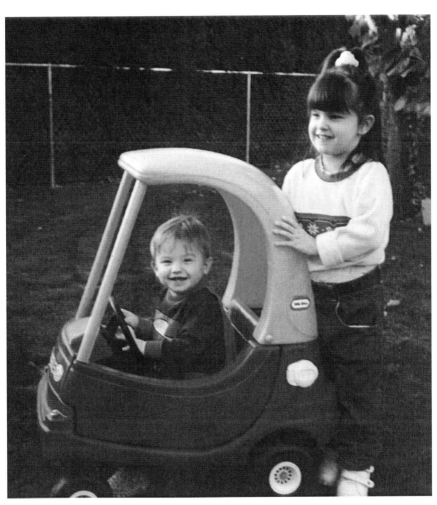

(Jesse giving Avery a helping hand)

Chapter 32
Time Flies By

June 26, 2011 (13 years later)

Thirteen years ago, I couldn't have imagined what life would be like for me in 2011, and wouldn't have wanted to try. I knew all too well the sudden curve balls life was capable of throwing at any given moment. Yet, here I am still in one piece, gratitude still intact, and in the process of transforming my journal into a book that I hope will inspire others to realize how fortunate they are, and to "seize the day."

Through our experience with Avery I've never lost sight of what was really important in life. Avery gave us many gifts, one being an immense sense of appreciation. I value life more than I ever have—not just life, but loving all those I hold dear to my heart. Still, whenever I think about how lucky I am, I begin to cry, because I can barely believe it. Over the years Avery has learned what my tears mean, and he calls them "happy tears."

As you can imagine, much has taken place these past twelve years. It's difficult to know where to begin my recap.

Cam and I have had the joy and privilege of watching our two babies grow and develop into wonderful, healthy, happy adolescents.

Avery is thirteen, and has turned into the most handsome young man. He looks so much like Cam, with his tall, slim physique and his ocean-blue eyes. Jesse, who is now sixteen, is as gorgeous as ever and still possesses the captivating presence she had when she was three. This hasn't always been the case though. Many of the past twelve years have been incredibly challenging for Jesse—as I'll explain in a moment.

Since Avery's last surgery, he's never looked back. Once his heart was fixed, he has been the easiest baby, aside from being a fussy eater. Really, if people would have looked in our window at feeding times, I'm certain they would have been mortified. Avery would be strapped into his highchair and many times I would distract him with cartoons while I shoved a spoonful of food in his mouth. Sometimes one feeding would take up to forty-five minutes. It was either that or have surgery to insert a feeding tube through his stomach. That wasn't an option.

Avery certainly kept Cam and I on our toes and had me wondering if Dr. LeBlanc had installed a bionic heart in him. Between the years of two and five we couldn't keep up. He had no fear and would literally swing off the light fixtures. Our house was locked up like Fort Knox because he was constantly trying to escape. If we went anywhere Cam and I had to take shifts watching him because if we let him out of sight for more than a few seconds, he was "gone like the wind." Our friends would get exhausted just watching us take turns chasing him all over the place. As exhausting as it was, I never complained too much because I was just happy he was there for me to chase.

On one particular holiday, however, I must have aged at least ten years. Avery was about two-and-a-half, and Jesse five, when we decided to spend a few days in a nice waterfront hotel in Kelowna for a mini-getaway and to visit our friends, Brent and Madonna. About 7:00 in the morning we heard Jesse making some funny noises and when we checked on her we realized that Avery was missing! Frantically screaming, we asked Jesse where Avery was. She pointed at the door to the hallway and said, "Out there."

Cam (in his underwear) and me (with pajamas on) raced out the door shouting Avery's name. Not knowing what time Jesse had opened the door for him, and especially because we were on the waterfront, I feared the worst. I felt emotionally and mentally paralyzed with no rational sense of what to do. Cam ran to the elevator and pressed the button, while I ran down the hallway hollering "Avery!" at the top of my lungs. I woke up everyone on the ninth floor. When the elevator door opened, there was Avery standing innocently with his heavy diaper hanging to his knees.

At that time, Jesse's vocabulary still wasn't great and the best we could decipher was that Avery had wanted to go on an adventure so Jesse had helped him on his quest. At this hotel there were no kid-proof latches at the top of the doors to keep them locked, so for the remainder of our stay the heavy couch was pushed up against the door at night.

Bonnie was right. She said most of "heart babies" grew up to be wonderful, well-adjusted kids. I had been a little worried she was wrong because Avery was so spoiled in his first few years. We were so happy he was here, nothing else mattered. On occasion I feared he would grow up to be a self-centered, spoiled brat. However, the opposite has occurred. Avery is the friendliest thirteen-year-old I've had the pleasure of knowing, with an immense loving and giving attitude. He goes out of his way to help people feel good, always speaking words of encouragement.

I seriously can't begin to count how many people tell me what a kind, generous, happy boy he is. Even at almost age thirteen, he must give me at least three or four hugs in one day as he tells me I'm the best mom in the world and that he loves me. I don't think I have the best parenting skills, but I do know that the enormous love and appreciation Cam and I provide is the best parenting skill we could have.

Avery's only setback is his fine and gross motor skills. The doctors describe it as a mild cerebral palsy, resulting in a slightly weakened right side, which causes some stiffness and imbalance. Avery certainly doesn't let this inhibit him in any way. Last year he missed A-honors by only one point, and played on all the sports teams until grade seven. I admire his perseverance in facing all his challenges. His CP causes some coordination and balance difficulties, and greatly inhibits his athletic ability, but this certainly doesn't stop him. Avery exhibits frustration sometimes, but he always gives 110 percent. He demonstrates to me every day that humans are born with strength of mind and will. The determination he showed at birth is every bit as evident now as it was then.

Every day since Avery was born he continues to captivate the hearts of all whose paths he crosses. A prime example was his grade six year during Sports Day. Everyone knew each other at Cheam Elementary because it's a small rural school consisting of around 130–150 students a year. Avery has gone to school with most of his peers since kindergarten, and they all knew his relentless persistence to keep up. Every year the teachers, parents, and children continued to see Avery struggle at Sports Day. Every year Avery returned with his desire to win the 100-meter sprint, only to again meet disappointment. This year was his last at elementary school and he was more determined than ever to win, but as he began to run he tripped and fell ... then lay motionless on the field.

Cam and I ran to see if he was okay, and found him physically fine. Just his ego had taken a bruising. He started to cry and was embarrassed to get up, but one of the other parents, Remmert Hinlopen, ran onto the field, scooped Avery up and finished the race with Avery on his shoulders. All the parents, teachers, and students loudly chanted, "Avery! Avery!" as they ran across the finish line. Tears filled my eyes, and as I looked around the track, I noticed the crowd full of emotion, with most wiping their eyes as well.

Avery set the bar very high for himself, thus causing frustration when he felt he had fallen short. Despite the positive support and reinforcement Cam and I provided, Avery often was too hard on himself. Even though it upset me to see him disappointed, I knew that this was his strong will manifesting itself—the same will that had enabled him to survive four heart surgeries. He was, and always will be, my biggest hero.

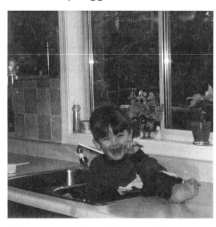 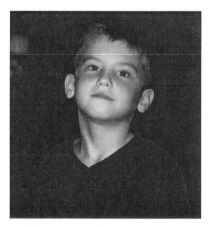

(*Avery brushing his teeth*)   (*Avery starting grade one*)

As I had anticipated, there were many bumps along the road for Jesse. When she was six years old, we finally got the diagnosis:

she was autistic. From the research I had done on my own, I'd already come to that conclusion. Unfortunately, we had to see many doctors before we could receive a formal diagnosis. Twelve years ago, many people hadn't even heard the word, let alone knew what it meant. Plus, Jesse was high functioning, making a diagnosis even more difficult.

Finding out Jesse had autism didn't really rattle me until years after the diagnosis. It wasn't the fact she had autism that was most difficult to deal with, it was the lack of support out there for families with autistic children—along with all the broken promises that new therapies brought.

Over the years we have gone through umpteen therapies with Jesse, from bio feedback treatments to chelation therapy, and many in between. Generally, the only result from any treatment was disappointment from *lack* of results. I was still the eternal optimist I had always been though. I would get my hopes up so high about a new treatment, only to have them dashed from a lack of success. I guess I'd rather have it that way than to go through life a skeptic.

Jesse is in grade ten now and able to participate in all of her academic and elective classes with the support of a teaching assistant. Everyone she meets adores her. She charms people with her outgoing enthusiasm and her zest for life. She has the amazing, gifted ability to see only the good in people and the wonderful things life has to offer. But she also harnesses an innate sixth sense, wishing to keep her distance from certain people.

It hasn't always been this way. Jesse's lack of ability to articulate her emotions and feelings has been the cause of much frustration and anguish for her. The years between eleven and fifteen brought many meltdowns along with some aggressive behavior at times. It made for challenging times in our family. Fortunately, I was always able to draw the strength to work through the difficult times, and continue to find new ways to help and support Jesse. It wasn't easy, and many times I pulled out my journal to remind myself of everything I had to be grateful for.

Last year was a particularly challenging time with Jesse for a couple of reasons. I was finally realizing after exhausting all my avenues that I couldn't "fix" her. I had always thought I would be able to cure Jesse, or at least come *close* to helping her with a cure to autism—primarily so she could feel more understood and carry less anxiety about being in a world where she felt so misunderstood.

As much as it was difficult to admit, I also wished to find a cure for my own selfish reasons: I wanted a daughter like all my friends had, one I could shop with, talk with, and one day watch walk down the aisle at her wedding. I started to grieve knowing that I would never share in her joy as she gave birth to her first child. It was such a difficult balance. On the one hand, I didn't want to place a ceiling on Jesse's abilities; but on the other, I wanted to be realistic about what her future held.

It broke my heart when Jesse reached Middle School and all her childhood friends went their own ways, disappearing from our lives. The birthday invitations stopped, along with the visits. This made me furious and I wanted to phone and scold all of Jesse's friends, or actually their parents. She was so social and loved people, and couldn't understand why her friends didn't want to hang out with her anymore. I was mad at their parents for not supporting their children's friendship with Jesse. After a short period of time I realized it was a waste of energy to stress about something I had no control over. I couldn't make people behave the way I would've, or make them do what I thought was right. It was their loss. After that, whenever I saw Jesse's old friends or their parents, I gave a big smile and held my head high with pride knowing I had a truly wonderful daughter.

It was a year that brought many realizations for me. It took some time, but thank goodness I came to know that Jesse didn't need to be fixed. She was happy and healthy, and that was all that mattered. I had and would continue to embrace her unique traits. Jesse was comprised of qualities that only parents with special needs children share the privilege of knowing. Jesse saw the good in all people, never holding a grudge. She displayed unconditional love. The littlest things would always please her, like the breeze she felt on her face while soaring back and forth on her Grandma's swing. If her day consisted of having made someone smile, she felt very successful.

There was no point in mourning who she would never be. I needed to celebrate who she was now. As humans we'll always have a choice, and it's a much richer life when we choose to find the "silver lining." There always is one. Sometimes, however, a person has to look deep to find it.

My second struggle last year was in December when Jesse had surgery on her back to correct her scoliosis (curvature of the spine). Her spine had curved to the point where it was putting pressure on her lungs. This was a major seven-hour surgery where the surgeons fused metal rods to Jesse's spine in order to straighten her back. This required a week's stay at Children's Hospital.

When I first heard this news I felt the old, familiar feeling of my world crumbling around me. Here we were going back to Children's Hospital, only with our other child this time. The months we had spent there with Avery felt fresh, and I began to feel myself becoming the same lost soul I had been twelve years earlier. My only choice was to press on like I had before with hope and belief in a positive outcome.

One of my biggest concerns was how Jesse would cope with the surgery and the subsequent pain, not to mention spending a week confined to a hospital bed. The rods needed time to set to her spine, and I was riddled with worries, especially concerned that she wouldn't follow the rules requiring her to remain still and not to sit up during that time.

The twelve years since I had last occupied the OR waiting room, when Avery had his last heart surgery, seemed like yesterday. I became haunted with terrifying memories, vividly remembering every emotion and feeling—from the rapid pounding of my heart, to my ability to almost detach myself from my body as a coping mechanism. Fortunately, this time paled in comparison to those stays at Children's Hospital. Surgery was successful, and we were very proud of how bravely Jesse handled her recovery. She listened to the nurses and followed their instructions without fail. We were feeling pretty lucky that things had gone so smoothly. We had dodged another bullet, or so we thought. Upon our return, home life continued to be what I liked to coin, "our normal." But then Jesse got a bad staff infection after her stitches came out. Cam and I took her to the doctor when we noticed that a small part of her incision looked like it hadn't sealed properly, and was oozing fluid.

The doctor set us up with an appointment at Chilliwack hospital with a wound nurse. Further tests confirmed that Jesse had a staff infection. Every three days we took her back to the hospital to get checked and to re-dress the wound. The dressing was lined with silver and special materials to draw the infection out. We also had Jesse on an oral antibiotic to help heal the infection. However, weeks later we still hadn't seen much improvement and expressed our concern. The wound nurse told us these infections take a long time to heal, and not to worry. Everything was going well.

Six weeks following surgery I drove into Vancouver with Jesse to meet Dr. Riley for a post-surgery checkup. Little did I know that I was about to get another shock of a lifetime. Dr. Riley nearly freaked out when he took Jesse's bandage off. He turned to me with a stunned expression and asked, "How long has it looked like this?"

I explained what happened following the removal of the stitches, and how we were seeing the wound nurse every three days to check and re-bandage the wound.

His voice took on an angry tone. "They should have sent you here a long time ago. This infection is really bad, and I need to schedule an emergency surgery to try to remove it. If the infection has reached the rods or the bone, surgery is blown and the rods will have to come out." Then he stormed out of the room.

I sat there in stunned disbelief, feeling more overwhelmed with each passing second. I fumbled for my phone and began to sob uncontrollably while I tried to make my fingers press the numbers of Cam's cell. I was nearly hyperventilating and barely coherent, and it took many breaths before I could attempt to explain to Cam what had just happened. When I finally succeeded, he was livid, calling the wound nurse some choice words. I told him I felt partly to blame because I had taken her word that she knew what she was doing. He said there had been no reason to doubt her; she had been confident the treatment was working, and she was a professional in wound treatment.

Seeing me upset triggered inconsolable sobbing in Jesse. Then I began to feel even worse. With much effort I managed to suppress my tears and comfort Jesse with hugs and tell her everything was going to be fine. I don't think she believed me, but it was enough to stop her from crying. Jesse kept saying, "I can't have another surgery. I can't go through this again."

I remembered my Dad telling me my dog Sam would be okay after he was nearly killed by a car. I took the same leap of faith and told her that she'd be just fine. I knew it was possibly not true, but at the time I needed to do all I could to give her some peace.

I was holding Jesse in my arms, with silent tears sneaking from my eyes, when Dr. Riley returned to tell me surgery would be this Friday, two days away. He'd had to bump another child's surgery to fit Jesse in. He could see the wreck I was, and tried to turn his voice from anger to optimism. In a softer tone he told me he would hopefully be able to remove all of the infection on Friday without the rods having to come out. It didn't matter what he said. I was devastated. He apologized for his abrupt behavior, and expressed his disappointment with the wound nurse from Chilliwack.

The drive back to Chilliwack was horrible. I probably shouldn't have been driving, but I just wanted to get home. I could barely retain my sanity but I tried to hold things together for Jesse's sake. She was terribly upset she had to have another surgery, and was refusing the idea altogether.

Finally, after two agonizing days, Friday arrived. This time surgery was only a couple hours of tortuous waiting, and fortunately our prayers were answered: the infection had not yet traveled to the bone or rods, and Dr. Riley was able to successfully remove all of the infection. What could have turned out disastrously turned into another blessing. Jesse recovered beautifully and now carries a nice straight posture.

For about a month following the surgery I fell back into a post-traumatic stress state. I couldn't understand: Jesse had ended up being okay, so why was I so depressed? I guess the effects of all our challenges these past thirteen years had surfaced. For a short period of time I wasn't my cheerful optimistic self and didn't really want to be around people. I felt deprived and deflated. Thankfully, the promise I had made to God found its way back into my soul, and I was able to regain my gratitude.

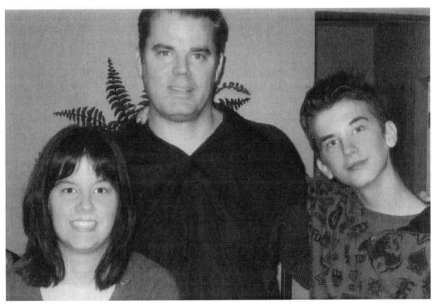

(2011: Jesse, Cam and Avery)

The plus side to dealing with so much adversity in life is the wonderful reward that we receive when we finally rise above it. All I had gained from Avery's experience wasn't lost after all, and returned in full force. I realize there will be more challenges ahead in my life, but I know I've obtained the fortitude to meet them head on. My mentor Napoleon Hill often said that with every adversity, a seed of its equivalent comes with it.

Cam is also one of the reasons I remain strong. We're still one great team, and I'm so proud of us. It's been close to twenty years, and within them we have had our ups and downs, but our love and respect for each other has always prevailed. When Joanne

Woodward was asked how she and Paul Newman had been able to make it together through fifty years in a Hollywood marriage her reply was, "I guess we were just lucky. We never fell out of love at the same time."

I have always been in love with Cam, and I'm sure that he felt the same way about me, but there had been times when we'd let our relationship nearly get lost in the shuffle. The obstacles that come with raising two children with challenges brought some hectic times, and it was easy to fall short in other important areas of life. Fortunately, Cam and I have been able to get back on track. Our love has endured many obstacles, and we have managed to rise above them.

A few years ago, Cam decided to switch careers and became a realtor. He was unhappy with the waste business, and had always had an interest in real estate. I was a little nervous about the transition, but I knew that life is too short to be doing something you no longer enjoy. Many people thought we were crazy, but at the end of the day we knew what really mattered. For a while it was tough and sometimes I joked to our friends we'd need to be standing in the food stamp line soon. However, I wasn't too worried; we had survived much worse. Fortunately, Cam is a natural at it and thoroughly enjoys going to work each day. I believe the biggest indicator of success in a person's career is if they enjoy what they do.

About twelve years ago I started a part-time business of my own. I do specialty painting, mostly working with plaster, doing textured walls, and granite finishes. I began restoring a lot of old fireplaces and painting feature walls in homes. I love doing it, and it provides a very flexible schedule. I usually work about two to three days a week. I also became have become diligent at exercising, working out five to six days a week. I find it is the best remedy to reduce stress and anxiety. Plus, I feel so good, and have much enthusiasm.

I surround myself with wonderful people and have reconnected with many childhood friends. A core group of seven of my friends began getting together usually around once a week. We call ourselves the Kindergarten Group because most of us have been friends since elementary school. We count on and depend on each other like sisters, venting our problems and celebrating our achievements. Rhonda and her husband Brian have a spacious second home about three hours east of Chilliwack, in Tulameen, so we girls try at least once a year for a week's retreat.

One of the girls is, of course, Tracee. I'm glad to still have her in my life. Nikcole is also part of the Kindergarten Club. I will never forget, and will forever cherish, her unconditional love and support during Avery's first year. She will always be one of my best friends.

One of my favorite people (and fellow Leo), Heather, is in the group also. We have gone to school together since we were kids, and have become much closer since the move back to Chilliwack. Heather's younger sister, Elaine, has also become a wonderful friend. She has a special needs son, Colton, who is close to Jesse's age. Sharing the experiences and challenges of having such a child provides a deep bond.

Another terrific friend I reconnected with was Rhonda. We've become closer than ever in the past few years, and usually not a day has gone by that I haven't talked to her. I couldn't begin to count the many times her support has helped me. She is a true-to-self person who calls a spade a spade, and I just love that about her. She has a big heart and goes out of her way to help people in very selfless ways.

A few years ago I was a bridesmaid at the wedding of one of my best friends, Sherri. We have known each other ever since she dated Steven in Junior High. It wasn't until about six years ago that we reconnected and become great friends.

I also reunited with one of my best friends, Madonna. We were great friends back in the Burnaby days before I was married. She's back living in her home town Kelowna with her fiancée, Tim. We try to get together at least a few times a year.

Bonnie was married for about nine years, but it never worked out. However, last year she reconnected to the boyfriend who had broken her heart twelve years ago. I guess it took him that long to realize he had let go of the best thing he could have ever had. She had always known he was her soul mate and had loved him all those years. Her eyes now display a happiness and peace that I rarely see in others.

Working at Children's Hospital for so many years finally took its toll on her, so she has a new job at an adult hospital in the catheter lab. She likes it because her stress level is way down. Since she's back together with her boyfriend, we see less of her, but I'll always consider her one of my dearest friends, a person whom I look up to and greatly admire. She still calls Avery her Little Monkey Man.

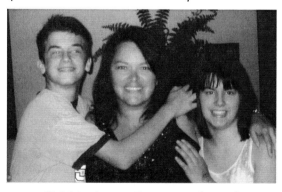

(2011: Avery, Bonnie and Jesse)

Over the years we've lost touch with Lisa and Ben. The last time we got together with them was when Avery and Tina were two. Eventually the phone calls became more infrequent until they stopped altogether. Even though I hear Tina is doing well and looks amazing on all her Facebook pictures, it must be difficult sometimes dealing with her cystic fibrosis. I know progress has been made, and hopefully with the continuous medical advances there will soon be a cure. From what I know of Tina, she's a fighter like Avery. I'm very proud of Lisa for doing an amazing job with her philanthropy work for Cystic Fibrosis. I'm not surprised. She has a lot of chutzpah.

Steven has had a bit of a rocky road following the end of my journal, but is back on his feet now. He and Tammy divorced about a year after Dad died. It wasn't too much of a surprise, and I think many could see it coming. Probably the easiest explanation would be to say they were childhood sweethearts who just slowly grew apart. Steven now has a great partner, Lorrie, whom he's been with for nine years. They have two gorgeous boys, Cole, nine, and Kade, seven. Over the years Lorrie and I have developed a close friendship. Cam and Steven are also very close, often getting together for a beer. Our families hang out together all the time, especially in camping season. We both have travel trailers and started camping in the spring and summer a few years ago. There is a group of between five to ten families that we camp with throughout the spring and summer.

I still see Tammy's mother, Heather. Since Chilliwack is a relatively small town we bump into each other every now and again. I often still think about the sacred message from God she gave me following Avery's birth.

Mom is doing better than ever and remains in the home Dad and she built over fifty years ago. She started exercising with me, losing about forty pounds, and looks terrific. A few years after Dad died, she took up golfing in the spring and summer, and curling in the winter. She has gone on a few dates over the years, but says there was no one who could come close to Dad. The two of us are as close as ever and even went on a Vegas trip together a couple years ago. It was so much fun that we decided that we'll definitely do it again. Every Sunday we still go to her house for supper, along with Steven, Lorrie, and the kids.

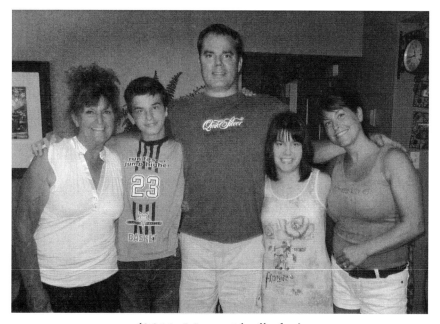

(2011: Mom with all of us)

Cam's dad Steve lost his lengthy battle to lung cancer in December of last year. This, of course, was a devastating loss to all of us. Cam was extremely close to his father, and took it very hard. It was difficult to see him in such emotional pain, but going through it myself, I knew it was only time that would ease the pain. Steve was seventy-seven when he passed away. It seems to me that no one is ever old enough to die, but at least Steve had lived a long, full life. He was able to spend many wonderful years watching his grandchildren grow up. Avery and Jesse were close to Papa, and are still close to Madge. She picks up the kids from school once a week to spend some time with them, and often baby-sits on weekends. We're pretty lucky because we get to also go there every Wednesday for dinner. Often Cam tears up as he thinks of the many wonderful memories he'd had with his dad.

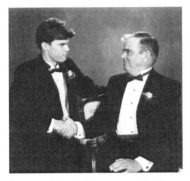

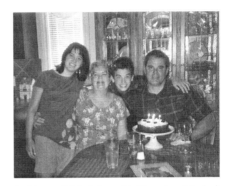

(Cam and his dad at our wedding)   (Avery's thirteenth birthday with Grandma Madge)

I still miss Grandma and Dad and think about them everyday, but the comfort of their presence is always close. It took three years but I was finally able to look at the one and only picture Mom took of Dad holding Avery. It was on a Sunday night when we were all over for supper. Up until then, I just hadn't been ready. For some reason, on this particular day, I wanted to see it.

After dinner I snuck into Mom's bedroom and opened the closet where she kept all the photo albums. It didn't take long to find the album I was looking for. I thumbed quickly through the pages until my eyes became fixated on the photo which will remain forever in my mind. There it was, the only picture I would ever have of the two of them together. Dad looked so proud, yet I could see his worry about Avery displayed in his eyes. It was difficult to look at it, and stirred many emotions along with some tears, but I'm glad that I finally did it. After a minute of reflecting, I quickly dried the tears, wiping away traces of smudged mascara, and blended back into the get-together as though nothing had happened.

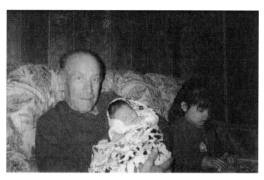

(The only photo of Dad and Avery five days before he passed away)

This year on Father's Day I was missing Dad a lot. It was a beautiful day and I was sitting outside enjoying the morning sun on my face, but as usual on Father's Day, feeling a little blue. I stared into the clouds, and with my eyes welling up into tears, for the first time ever, I asked my Dad to give me a message that he was still here with me. Later that day, I forgot about my request and was outside watching the kids play while Cam set up the new trampoline. Cam took a break to come and sit with me for a bit. We were talking, when all of a sudden I looked down to the ground, and staring up at me like it was a foot high off the ground was a four-leaf clover!

I said, "It can't be!"

"What?" Cam asked.

I walked a few feet from where I was, bent down and plucked it from the ground. From head to toe my body tingled with awe as I realized Dad had fulfilled my wish. This was my sign. I then told Cam how I had been feeling in the morning, and what I had asked my Dad.

Tears filled both our eyes as we embraced. It was a magical moment. My Dad is still with me, watching over and protecting me. I know it as sure as I'm sitting here now. There isn't a better comfort in the world.

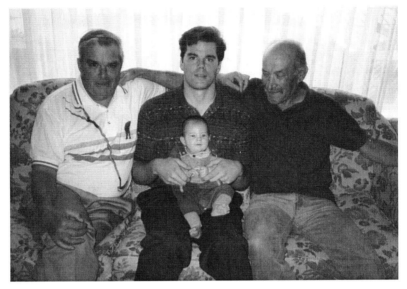

(Steve, Cam, Jesse and Dad celebrating Cam's first Father's Day)

I still find many four-leaf clovers on my life's path. They are pressed inside books all over the house. The other day raised the biggest goosebumps on my arms. It was a warm spring day and I decided to go on a run. As I was jogging down Williams Road, I stopped to take a break alongside my grandma's sisters' old house, where I had often gone with Grandma. One of my favorite songs, *Don't Stop Believing*, was playing on my mp3 player, and as my eyes gazed at the side of the road, what did I see? Yes indeed! It was a four-leaf clover staring right at me. I raised my head to the sky, feeling the warmth of the sun, smiled to the heavens and said a big "thank-you" to all those whose love and support continued to fill my life.

Thirteen years ago, I couldn't have guessed things would have turned out this way. I wouldn't say it was like those fictional story books where the princess and the prince live happily ever after, but it was close enough for me. Every day I think about having been blessed with Avery for twelve years—and hopefully I will have at least fifty more years here to spend with him.

As well, thirteen years ago I never would have imagined writing this book. Actually, writing a book was something I thought I would never do. I feel it's important to say: "Never, ever, *not* do something because someone said you couldn't, or that you weren't good enough." I say this because back in university, my second year English professor basically said that I couldn't write my way out of a wet paper bag. Well, it sure is a good thing I didn't listen to him, although I almost did.

When the persistent desire to tell my story never eased, I thought, "Well, how can I do that? I can't write." So I sought out a ghostwriter, but that cost way too much money, plus how could someone else tell my story with such compassion and conviction? It's my story, I lived it. So I faced my fears and sat down in front of the computer and allowed my fingers to effortlessly dance upon the keys to tell my story. Well, not always effortlessly. Many times I couldn't see the keys through the tears—tears that relived some pretty hard times of my life, but also the most rewarding. Sometimes it took an hour to write one small paragraph. Often I would find inspiration to write at the oddest times, like camping with friends and family for instance.

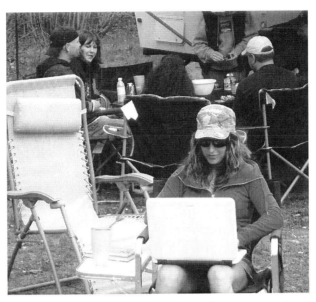

(Writing Bravery on laptop while camping)

No matter what your situation, whether your teacher thinks you're wasting desk space, or you have a less-than-encouraging parent, or a partner who makes you feel less than capable, never let them discourage you from doing anything you wish to accomplish. Just give it a try and you may be surprised. It's important to know: the only person who can tell you what you can or can't do is yourself. My mom was right when she spoke those words to me forty years ago on my first day of kindergarten when I said I couldn't do it. She said, "Kimmi, there is no such word as *can't*." Thank God for my mom.

Yes, there are times I feel a little shortchanged, but not many, and never for long. You see, I believe we have a choice with how we see our life, no matter what cards have been dealt to us. I can't change the cards God gave me. I can only be grateful He gave me any at all. My children are healthy and happy, and at the end of the day, what more can a parent want? I said twelve years ago in my journal: "I saw many parents leave the hospital without their babies. I was one of the lucky ones because mine got to come home with me." I don't need to dig deep into my soul to remember this. I feel it every day.

Avery and Jesse have taught me so much in their first years of life, yet very different lessons. Avery has provided me with an incredible sense of value, appreciation, and the intensity of love's bond. Jesse has allowed unconditional love to enter my heart, along with tolerance and acceptance.

I still often think back to the promise I made when Avery was in the hospital: "If Avery lives, and I get to take my baby boy home, I'll be the happiest mom on earth." Well, the feeling of bringing Avery home on that Thanksgiving Day twelve years ago still lives strong within me. Although there have been struggles along the way, I have honored my promise. When I find myself having a bad day, I close my eyes and relive the feeling of that miraculous Thanksgiving Day ... and it doesn't take long for gratefulness to return. And all is well in my world again.

THE POEM BONNIE WROTE FOR AVERY ON HIS FIRST BIRTHDAY

MAY 29, 1999

To my Little Monkey Man, Avery

There was no gift that I could give you on this, your first and very special birthday,

That would even come close to expressing what a special boy you are to not only me,

But to all whose lives you have touched. That was why I have written you this letter.

When many more birthdays have passed and you have become a man, I hope that if

You still have this letter you will always know how much love you have brought to my

Life.

It was hard to imagine that one year ago you were so tiny. To look at you now with so

Many smiles and so much spirit it is hard to believe how many times we came so

Close to losing you. Thank God for watching you so closely. Thank God for giving you

The parents, sister, and grandparents that

you have who loved you into living.

Birthdays are a time of gift giving and I want you to know that you Avery are our gift.

You've taught all of us all about strength, all about love, all about fear, and all

About life. How special that you have given so much wisdom in the first and

Miraculous year of your life.

As years pass, the memories of the difficult times of the past year will never leave

Us, but they will fade. The wonderful memories will however always leave a bright

Spot on our hearts. Life has a funny way of doing that - aren't we lucky! You, Avery,

Will never remember all that you endured in this first year as actual memories, but

The courage and strength will last forever. These are the gifts that you were born

With and for that, I am glad.

I am so happy to be celebrating this very special birthday with you and all who love

You. You are a treasure, Little Monkey Man,

and always remember... I love you.

Happy Birthday Avery

Love always,

Bonnie

AVERY'S HOMEMADE MOTHERS' DAY CARD TO ME IN GRADE THREE

Mom, you are so special to me and I want to share my favorite memories with you.

You took care of me when I was sick and you put a cold cloth on my forehead. Remember when you and I set up a surprise party for Dad. It made me very happy to help.

Remember when I took a big bite of my hot dog and the wiener slipped in my mouth and I was choking. You knew I was choking and you grabbed the wiener out of my mouth and you saved my life. I was the happiest and luckiest boy, and you were a super hero.

Love, Avery

AVERY'S POEM HE WROTE IN GRADE FIVE

If I were in charge of the world,

I'd cancel all name calling, and I'd make the Incredible Hulk the movie for toddlers.

If I were in charge of the world,

There would be lots of hovercrafts, and kids would be allowed to have swords.

If I were in charge of the world,

You wouldn't have backstabbing kids.

You wouldn't have rude people.

You wouldn't have homework or evil people.

If I were om charge of the world,

Blue bubblegum ice cream would be a vegetable, and all horror movies would be "G".

And a person who sometimes forgot to bring his stuff, and sometimes forgot his identity, would still be allowed to be in charge of the world.

Jesse's English Essay, grade nine

My Invention

Nice Machine

Sometimes people are not very nice to each other.

I would like to help people be nice to each other.

My machine is a Be A Good Friend Machine.

The machine will kiss them if someone is hurt, Or if they are being mean.

A person will go to the machine that was in the Loving Garden where the flowers are.

The machine will give you flowers to make you feel better.

The machine also gives hugs.

The Be a Good Friend Machine is really tiny, And we can go on it together.

I would have a lot more friends if I had this machine.

Jesse

Acknowledgments

The notion that I wrote a book still shocks me. Not just any book, but a special book that has already touched the hearts of so many, and hopefully many more to come. My wish is to help comfort families going through adversity, and invoke gratitude in all parents of children.

It's difficult to know where to begin my acknowledgments; there are so many incredible people in my life that have helped me become who I am, and supported me throughout such turbulent times. You will come to know them very well during the reading of this book.

Mom, Dad, and Grandma, thank you for all the unconditional love and encouragement you provided to me through the years. Your love for me fostered the belief that I could do anything I set my heart to. I am blessed to have been under your wings, protected and guided through this unpredictable and sometimes challenging world. You provided me with the strength to rise above adversity with grace and pride.

Avery and Jesse, thank you for gracing me with your presence and coming into the world as my children. Your time here has taught me more about life and living than any amount of schooling ever could. You have humbled me, and made me a better person. Being your mother has allowed me to feel the full capacity love bestows.

Cam, thank you for all your understanding and support. I couldn't have made it through these harrowing times without you. We have been an amazing team. I believe what we have been through together would have broken many. Thanks for hanging in there with me; I always knew you were special.

Steven, although you are my little brother by four years, you feel like my big brother, one who would protect his sister at any cost. You are a comfort to me that words cannot describe.

Bonnie, thank you for all your passionate care for Avery, and the support and friendship you provided to me. You are the best nurse I know and a trusted and valued friend. You went above and beyond your duty with Avery, and I felt a comfort when he was on your watch.

Nikcole, you were a pillar for me, who was wholeheartedly there for me and my family throughout this crisis. You gave up so much of your time to be with me, and stayed strong for me during my weak moments. Through the years, and still today, I know you will always be there for me. Thank you so much.

Dr Human, I don't even know what to say to you; articulating any words of my gratitude escapes me. For many months you gave me hope when there was none. I could see your passion and determination that Avery would survive. It wasn't just a job for you. We were real people, with real emotions, and you treated us so carefully and gently. Thank you so very much for making our devastating months spent at Children's Hospital a little less painful.

Dr. LeBlanc, you will always remain larger than life in my mind. I am in awe of how you carried the responsibility of all your precious little heart patients in your hands. Sometimes you carried the weight of the world on your shoulders, yet you remained steadfast in your duty. I always felt Avery was in the best hands with you; this means everything to a parent enduring a crisis.

Elaine, Heather, Madonna, Rhonda, and Tracee, thank you for all the times you dropped everything to come to my aid during the trying times I have endured. Your comfort and support helped me to rebuild the strength to overcome many adversities. Tracee, I am grateful for all your enthusiastic excitement towards Bravery, along with cheering me on to follow my dreams. Your encouragement filled me with positive energy.

I am indebted to all my family and friends for your support through the challenging years, and for the encouragement to write this book. There are too many to list, but you know who you are.

Thank you to all the readers who picked up my book. I am honored to be sharing my story. I will be donating some of the proceeds to important children's charities. I hope Bravery will touch you in some way, and that you take away something valuable from it.